Larry's Way

By the Author of

Show Me the Way to go Home

Larry's Way

Larry's Way

◆

ANOTHER LOOK AT ALZHEIMER'S FROM THE INSIDE

Larry Rose

iUniverse, Inc.
New York Lincoln Shanghai

Larry's Way
ANOTHER LOOK AT ALZHEIMER'S FROM THE INSIDE

iUniverse, Inc.

For information address:
iUniverse, Inc.
2021 Pine Lake Road, Suite 100
Lincoln, NE 68512
www.iuniverse.com

ISBN: 0-595-28927-4

Printed in the United States of America

Contents

Acknowledgments

Jo Ann Davenport
Jacqueline Parris
Mae Belle Minerich
Sharon McGee
Stella Guidry
Marsha Arabie
Mary Lockhart
My Sisters Lois and Elsie

All who have given me encouragement to write this book.
More than they will ever know.

Foreword

Larry Rose's second book offers a unique reflection of the rate of progression of Alzheimer's disease in this very special individual. Compare to his first book. Show Me The Way Home, this reader come away with a roller coaster sensation of haunting feelings. The writer was sometimes angry, often frustrated, occasionally acerbic and at time morbid, but always a sense of serenity is pervasive to reassure us that this dreaded Alzheimer's is not going to take away one thing that Larry values most, his dignity. It is unusual for Alzheimer's patients to write well if at all; losing the ability to register and recall recent memory makes Larry Rose an ultimate existentialist whose writing should be read by all who are involved in the care of victims of Alzheimer's disease.

Pham H. Liem, MD
Medical Director, Center for Alzheimer's and related disorders
University of Arkansas for Medical Sciences

Preface

This book is about Alzheimer's in general and about my struggle in particular. It is written to put people in touch with the reality of a disease not read about widely in the ordinary course of life.

The purpose of this book, second in a series, depicts real people, real events, in the real world of an Alzheimer's patient.

As you read this book, the reader must judge for himself how well I have turned these unexplainable thoughts into printed words. You will judge favorably, I hope.

My address: Larry Rose
               Box 1411
               Fairfield Bay, Ar. 72088

Larry

1

Like A Fish Bowl

It is been three or four years now, maybe longer, since I was first diagnosed with Alzheimer's disease. Another two or three years before that, I first began exhibiting signs of this nefarious disease. It is understood that in the past five years, or so, my life has been somewhat different. I have had days, even months that life was normal, at least to me. Days when you feel like talking to the neighbors, mowing the lawn or listening to the golden oldies on the radio.

There are other days when I feel that with death or a nursing home so close, so ever present, what is the use of struggling any longer? How can I win? How can any of us, with this thing in our heads, win against this remorseless fusillade?

When you feel like a whole person, you are in control of yourself and of your surroundings. I don't have that feeling of control any longer. Is it forgotten? If there is a spark of that feeling left, it is almost unreachable for me. It is like having your head in a fish bowl. You can see out, but nothing can get in.

My father always taught me to go as far in life as my own limitations will allow, each day further than the last. Now, to me, there is no future, no past. I am trapped in this dull numbing present. I have to face the fact and accept what has happened to me and to resign myself to the certainty that I will soon be at the end of this wonderful life. I sometimes think that this is all a bad dream and that I will wake up soon and it will all be gone. That I will be the old "Larry" again. When I am forced to face reality, it is still there and it never goes away. I can face the end. It really does not bother me that much and, of course, I can't change it. No one can. I just can't accept it.

I can face what happened to me because; I think it was caused by fate. Pure chance. Almost all of the dreaded diseases that I can think of, with a few exceptions, can be prevented with a little precaution, or treated aggressively with some sort of medication. We all know by now that some types of lung cancer can be prevented by not smoking. Watch that fatty food to prevent heart problems and cholesterol buildup that can cause strokes, blocked arteries and the like. A person

1

has at least a little control over those diseases. I wish someone would tell me how in the hell you could prevent Alzheimer's. Contracting Alzheimer's, like MD, or MS, has got to be just the luck of the draw. One has no control over chance. You just play with the cards that are dealt to you. Like in the Kenny Rogers song, "You got to know when to hold em and know when to fold em".

Somehow the world keeps on turning without my help. The Dow is hanging in around 9,000; it seems to set a new record high almost every day. The market seems to be standing on its own two feet without any help from me. One wonders what he or she has contributed to the world during his or her lifetime. Does anyone ever make a lasting contribution? Abe Lincoln, perhaps. Generations from now, will anyone even care that I once lived here? That I walked the Ozarks, smelled the flowers?

Although most of my friends are of real support for me, with encouragement to keep doing all I can, there are always a few that never miss an opportunity to ridicule and to show how smart and astute they are. Such an incident happened just the other morning at my favorite hang out, "Mel's Diner". I had just finished having my usual morning coffee with all of my café cronies, when an acquaintance, I won't call him a friend, stopped me as I was leaving.

"Hi Larry, How are things? I haven't seen you for a while."

"I have been well, at least until the last few days," I said, as we chatted for a moment. I have been fighting this cold that everyone is catching right now."

"Is there an echo in here?" he said, "You have already told me that three time in the last minutes." Was he joking with me? Trying to get my goat? I couldn't tell. I don't remember repeating myself. I was visibly upset.

One of the waitresses that was standing nearby said, "Don't let him get to you, Larry. He doesn't understand."

"It's OK sweetheart, I won't let him get to me. One can't take serious anyone that thinks "Moby Dick" is a Venereal Disease," I said for everyone at the counter to hear. I went on home.

I try to tell myself that things like that don't bother me, but that would not be true. It does. I have tried to live my whole life without ever hurting anyone's feelings, but unfortunately, I am changing my attitude with Asses like that. As long as I can still think and talk, I refuse to become a minion, an obsequious follower or subordinate agent to someone's sick ego.

2

Good Friends

Stella Guidry is my caregiver, counselor, guardian, CPA, and best friend. It would be difficult indeed to go on without her help. She is a sweet, loving, caring person and a twenty-one karat Cajun, as the locals call themselves. When I get down in the dumps, just looking at her makes me feel better. She has those eyes that reach out and touch. She always has a good word for me. She cares. She can tell my mood just by looking at me.

You look like you could use a hug." She might say, "I can see that you are upset."

Praise, encouragement and a show of affection can go a long way in calming an Alzheimer patient. I can tell you from experience. It can be very upsetting, even frightening when I am speaking to someone that does not speak clearly or does not use direct sentences, uses slang, is unwilling to repeat and does not use a tone of voice that is warm and empathetic. I know this is asking a lot from someone that is not affected or is not used to talking to an Alzheimer's patient, but that is the purpose of these writings; to let folks know how it feels to be on this side. Please don't talk in abstract. Get the patient's attention and then ask simple questions. Avoid contradiction or arguing, if possible. It will only make the person more upset.

With Stella, I don't have to say a word to be understood. I can't say enough about Stella. She has an uncanny ability to sense what I am thinking and answer or act accordingly. A truly remarkable person with an inner beauty that no one who knows her can deny. Some misunderstand her because they don't know her. If it is facts and figures you want, she can help you. If it is BS you are after, you just had a bad day. She won't say a word until you ask her a question and only then will she tell you exactly what she thinks. Good or bad. But, when the chips are down, you can always count on her for help.

It has always amazed me how people in different parts of the country treat me so differently. I wrote earlier about some of the things that have happened to me.

I run across someone always every day that has some smart assed thing to say. Not so in the hill country of Arkansas. (There is one exception, The Fairfield Bay Community Club,) I will explain them later.

My place is in the Ozark Mountains. I have a cabin there. Stella and I once spent much time there, before this illness and even during the early stages. I don't get there too often anymore, much to my regret. It is a beautiful place, set high on a mountain and in a coppice of Oak and Hickory trees. There is a creek with a waterfall at the bottom of the property. A good place to sit and think. I fall in love with it all over again every time I go there.

Although the place is far back in the woods, I have some neighbors that are close by. Bonnie Brannon is one of them. Bonnie is a giant of a man. He has broad shoulders and a broad smile. He must be near seven feet tall with mighty muscles. Two hundred fifty pounds, not an ounce of fat. He is well over seventy years old by now. He is an affable man that gives new meaning to the word gentleman. His old blue eyes are the eyes of an honest man.

Many an evening he and I would sit talking on my front porch and watch the sun go down behind the ridge to the west. I would listen to the man tell tales of the old days when he was a boy. Coon hunting, logging, etc., I could go on and on. Far into the night I would sit patiently listening to him talk and the night creatures would come out with their usual noises, lightning bugs lighting the area around the meadow in front of the cabin.

Floyd, my pet "Pot Belly" pig, would sit with us. On occasion, he would get up and go out into the meadow and root up something good to eat, perhaps a truffle, then come back, oink a time or two, then lay down at our feet and go to sleep, his tail wagging all the time. He is one happy pig.

When the stars and moon come out, up there on the mount, it seems they are ten times brighter than anywhere near the cities. Sometimes it looks like the moon could get stuck in the treetops. I just love it. I think it is impossible to have stress in your life when one is able to spend a week or two in that place.

As Bonnie would leave to walk back down the trail to his cabin, I would sit alone for a while and think. "Anyone seeing this gentle giant walking down the trail, especially when Floyd would walk along with him for a time, would have to turn for a second look, such sights are seldom seen."

For years, Bonnie and I were the only ones on the mountain. Bonnie would spend hours with me, walking through the woods, showing me different kinds of plants. I have learned a lot from Bonnie. For a man with little or no education, he can sure teach a person a lot about the mountains.

"This one is good for Poison Ivy," he would say. "You just rub it together in your hands and make kind of a paste, then rub it on the places where it itches and the itch will go away. This one is called Penny Royal. You take a few of the little plants and boil it down in a bit of water and make a tea. Drink the tea slowly. Take an hour if you want. The Ticks won't get on you for a year. There is a plant here called Ginseng. It is hard to find but it is good for a lot of ailment. You will learn how to use it. Never pull it all. Save some for seed so it will come back next year. This is Poison Ivy. If you see this in the woods, don't wipe your ass with it." He laughed.

Bobby McGee and his wife, Sharon, were the next neighbors to come to the mountain. He bought some land down the mountain behind Bonnie's cabin. They have been there a couple of years by now. Bobby is an equally nice fellow; He and his wife are always willing to help the neighbors when the need arises. The McGee's have a lot of stuff. If you ever need to borrow something, they have it.

Also in the area is the Dean Thomas family. They live down the mountain on the trail out to the highway. He and his wife Karen, and a couple of teenagers moved into an old house that had been there for many years. They fixed it up and continue to work on the place all of the time, planting fruit trees, flowers and the like. It is really shaping up to be a nice place. On some nice mornings, I walk down there and have coffee with them while sitting around a table on their back porch. We chat about everything happening in the world and listen to Sid's call in show on the local radio station. It is a show where you can call in and buy or sell things that you don't need anymore.

All of these mountaineers are good, honest, hard-working people and over time have eased their way into my heart and mind. They know all about my illness and go out of their way to make sure I am all right while I am there alone. If they don't see me around for a period of time, one of them will come to see about me. I would like to think that I have eased my way into their hearts as well.

Unlike my home in Louisiana, not-with-standing my close friends, folks that live in the Ozarks treat me a lot differently. I have met and talked to a lot of different people there and never once did any one of them say anything to make me feel uncomfortable. On the contrary, they help by saying, "This is the right amount of change." One day I had occasion to transact some business at the accounting office at the Country Club in Fairfield Bay. The lady that I talked with there was not long in detecting that I had a problem. The name on her desk suggested her name was Pam Hilger.

"You appear to have some sort of affliction, Larry, It is something you can talk about?" she asked.

"I don't mind at all. I think the Doctors call it Alzheimer's disease." I stated.

She smiled. "Talk to me Larry, I have heard about it but I have never met anyone with this disease."

We talked for a long time. She listened intently; asking a question from time to time It was nearing the lunch hour when she asked. "Would you like to go out and have something to eat? We can continue our conversation."

"Sure, I would like that very much," I replied.

"I would too, Let's run over to the club, they are having Potato Soup for lunch today, Please be my guest," she stated with the usual smile.

"I insist on paying." I said.

"No way. You are my guest, she said firmly.

"You talked me into it. I am glad you are not selling Buick's. I may show up here everyday at about this time." I said smiling.

She didn't answer, just smiled back.

It was about a mile from her office to the golf course and restaurant so it was necessary to drive. "My truck is parked over there." I said, pointing to the truck.

"My car is closer. Just right here, Get in."

I got into her car and continued our conversation as she drove. I wasn't paying any attention to where she was going when we left the parking lot, I was talking when I should have been watching where we were going. It is very important to me that I know exactly where I am at every moment. If I have the feeling of being lost. I start to panic. She was taking a different route than I do and suddenly I was in strange surroundings. I could hardly take it.

Stop Pam, you are going to have to go back to the parking lot."

"Did you forget something?"

"No. I am lost."

"Oh, don't worry, I am going to bring you back." She said.

"No! You don't understand, I don't know where I am. I must go back to my truck to get straightened out." She slowed to turn around when I recognized the fire station. "I know where I am now, Pam, it's okay."

The damage was done. When I panic like that, I don't do anything right for a time. I can't talk, or walk. It is like this thing is my head is spinning out of control.

We drove on, with her pointing out where she lived, some of the churches, etc. finally we got to the Club. As we went inside and was seated at our table, I said. "This must be frustrating for you, having to put up with my little quirks."

"Not as frustrating as it is for you, I am sure," She stated with her usual smile.

During lunch, I told her about Stella, Floyd, the Cabin and all of the other important things in my life and I heard about hers as well.

"You and Stella must come to my house for dinner someday when she is here with you." she said. "You have told me so many good things about Stella, I have just got to meet her. I would also like for you both to meet my husband, Jerry."

"We will take you up on that offer, I get. The very next time she is here."

The dinner plans settled, the conversation moved back to Alzheimer's. "Are you optimistic about your future?" she asked.

"Not at all, In fact I am worried as hell. I keep waiting for the other shoe to fall. Some of the patients that I met two years ago that were better off than I, are dead now, or in a nursing home. I just don't understand. I need a victory, even a small one, to keep me going. I don't understand this thing at all."

"It may be that you have a type that is somewhat different."

"I have thought of that as well, but I have learned not to ask a doctor if he is sure that I have Alzheimer's. They immediately tell me I am in denial and that I should have counseling. I quit asking." I said.

We finished lunch, drove back to the parking lot to my truck, said our good byes and I drove back to the cabin. I was happy to have met someone so understanding. I know that I live in a special world that not many know or understand or care, really...in my view. Because they don't know or understand, they fancy themselves wiser than I. I am not going to get into a war with anyone about who is wiser than whom. What does it matter anyway? It just seems to me that when someone stops to smell the flowers or stand for a moment to admire the beauty of the trees and mountains, you are called a dreamer or a fool. I am both.

I spend hours examining the cabin and marveling that I own it and that I built it myself. There is such a peaceful atmosphere here; it would be hard to be disquieted or fearful. For a patient or caregiver, there is nothing in the world that will relieve stress better than spending a week or two at a place like mine. If you don't have a cabin in the woods, get one, rent one, borrow one, or if you can afford it, buy one. DO IT. Your life will be more peaceful, I guarantee.

Anything one enjoys doing can relieve the stress, whether it is the cabin, fishing, hunting, golf, photography or just having a pig for a pet. Experiment. See what works for you. I just finished planting a couple of rows of corn in the meadow for the deer and coon to eat. I know that I will spend hours watching them when the corn is ready. Just this afternoon I caught two doe deer with my video camera as they were laying in the meadow. I love it. I watch it over and over.

I don't mean to dwell on the cabin, but it means more to me than anyone will ever know. Any stranger could tell that it is a man's cabin at a glance; the wooden beams, the cast iron wood stove, the loft and of course, the arrangement of the furniture. Everything is arranged for comfort and convenience with little regard to popular taste. I am alone here for a few days at a time, however I am rarely lonely. There are no splendid meals cooked here anymore, but I do keep a good supply of junk food. I usually gain a few pounds every time I am here.

If I don't watch myself, I find myself thinking about the future. I have to stop and tell myself that there is no point in dwelling on what might happen a year from now or what might not. I know down deep in my heart that I have something in my head that is eventually going to kill me. I know that there is less of "Larry" today than there was yesterday and there will be even less of me tomorrow. They tell me that this disease is progressive and certain; I personally don't believe in certainty. I have come to believe that certainty is impossible and that probability suffices to govern faith and practice. I must not let myself worry about tomorrow, just try to get through today. Worry does not do my head any good. Time is my worst enemy. Can't waste any.

At sometime in our lives, I think we have all wished on a star or dreamed of finding a genie in a bottle, or a fairy godmother or some such thing that would grant us a wish. I think if such a thing were possible, I would not wish for wealth or even health, but I would never have to leave this place. These hills, bluffs, rocks and rivers are not lifeless things to me. They live and breathe, laugh and cry as I do. I feel that when I leave this place, my last contact with my world will be broken. The only thing left on the earth for me is happening today, this minute, now. There is no yesterday and there may not be a tomorrow. I feel compelled to write about my feelings, my experiences, my fears and frustrations. Maybe someday the world will care about how an Alzheimer's patient copes. Maybe it will cause a caregiver somewhere how to better understand their loved one and to better understand their fears and frustrations.

I don't have any visions of becoming a Nobel Laureate and I doubt if my writings will have Stephen King working for wages. I wrote for the above reasons, also the Doctors think it is good therapy for me.

3

Memories

I have thought so much about memory since I became afflicted with Alzheimer's. There are so many things that stick in your memory for your whole life. Take for an example your first day of school, your first date, your first kiss or perhaps some decision that you made years ago that changed your life forever. A full moon perhaps or the smell of the pines in a wet forest. You can call on these memories at any time you want, but you never do. The memories are there at any time you want to retrieve them, and faster than any computer, but years go by and you rarely do.

Thinking back, I can recall every word that was said in my family for the entire day of December 7, 1941. I was four years old. It was cold that morning in western Kansas. My dad had taken my sisters to church, my brother was out hunting and my mother was cooking dinner. I remember dad coming into the house and stating that the Japs were bombing Pearl Harbor. I had never heard the word "Japs" mentioned in our house before or Pear Harbor either. I did not know what these words meant. I had no idea what was going on, but I can remember all that and that everyone was upset. What good are memories like that? I don't need them. I never use them. Ever.

I think it would be possible that one could literally forget half of everything he or she knows and never know the difference. Could be that something happens that you remember your first day of school or some such thing. It would only be for a fleeting moment and then you put it away for another ten years or so. Those kinds of memories are of little use to me. I would rather remember how to get to the post office. I am not saying that all old memories are not important. You can't live without some memories, i.e. fire is hot. You can't breathe underwater, you don't step out in front of a truck etc.

I know that sometimes I don't act "normal", but I don't think of myself as abnormal. I have read and I have heard folks say that Alzheimer's patients become mean and sometimes violent and my use foul language. I fight doing this as hard as I can. Why is it that when you can't think of the words you want to use in a sentence, you can always think of the four letter words? I just make a conscious effort not to use them. Sometimes I think some people push me to this limit just to see how I will react. I don't know. It seems that way to me. Yesterday I went to Wards to buy a new VCR. Stella's old one had burned up again. This makes the third time in as many years. Stella did not want to get it fixed again. Each time it costs about a hundred and thirty dollars to get it repaired. What with the price of the newer model, it is just not worth fixing anymore.

"Stell, I saw in the paper where we can buy a new one at Wards for around a hundred and forty bucks. At that price, if it lasts a year, we can just toss it and buy another new one. We will be money ahead. Let me go and see what I can find."

I was at the Wards store looking at the new VCRs. They were aligned with a juxtaposition that led me to believe that the stock person had little else to do. There were boldly printed price tags on every one. It would have been a boon to any shopper but me. The numbers were starting to confuse me. The confusion must have been showing on my face. One of the salesmen asked if he could help me. Could it be that he held a master's degree in physiognomy?

"Yes, I am looking for the cheapest VCR that you have." I said.

"This one is the one we sell the most of," he said, pointing at one of the machines. He was showing no enthusiasm at all.

"Is this the cheapest one you have?" I asked.

"This one is our best sellers," he stated.

"I thought I asked to see the cheapest one you have. One of us needs to study our listening skills." I said starting to ire.

"This one is our best seller," he stated again.

"It is becoming obvious that you had rather miss a sale than for me not to play your silly game. I think I will go somewhere that a salesman will listen to me and sell me what I want. And, I don't think I want to do business with anyone that ends a sentence in a preposition."

He didn't seem to care. He just turned and walked away. Is it me or just that this guy didn't know me? I must have seemed spurious to him or at least incongruous to the normal. It is what I expect anymore. With an attitude like that, I don't know how the man sells anything. He could not have worked for me ten minutes. If all of Ward's salesmen are like him, the stores could go belly up!

I drove on to Circuit City where I should have gone in the first place. There I met a young black salesman. I think I must have been his first customer ever. I told him exactly what I wanted. He picked it out for me and I bought it. One hundred and thirty bucks. It works just fine and it is not hard to program.

4

Medication

All my life I have tried to be salubrious. Not to any extreme, but at least generally. I don't drink or take drugs that are not prescribed. I try to eat right, exercise and do what most would say in promoting health. I do smoke a pipe now and then when I get nervous. It helps, in fact one of the Doctors in Little Rock told me to throw away the Ativan. He said, "I know, it is a hell of a thing for a Doctor to say, but the pipe will do you less harm that the drug."

We have all learned that our former President, Ronald Reagan, has been diagnosed with Alzheimer's I was saddened to learn of his plight. It does seem ironic that this same man that was so against fetal brain transplant research is now in a position that such research might have resulted in a cure for him…and me. In my view, to mix politics and research science is tantamount to book burning.

It seems every time I get optimistic about something positive in Alzheimer's research, government steps in and says "NO", you cannot do that! I have been participating in a new Drug study program at Ochsners Hospital in New Orleans. It has been going on for a couple of years. I can't say for sure that it has helped me, but I think it has and that is what matters most to me. I know that I can talk better than I could before I started the Program.

The study has been over for some time now. Consequently, the medication has stopped. There is what is called a "License for Compassionate Use", that will allow the Pharmaceutical company to continue to supply me with the medicine, but of course, our old friend and protector, the Government, namely the FDA, are dragging their feet in issuing the Compassionate use license. God only know when they will get around to doing that. In the meantime, a medication that I think was working well for me is not available under any circumstance. My government is protecting me to death. Like Shakespeare said, "Upon what meat are these Caesar's fed that they grow so great."

5

Affects

At some point in your life, before you are diagnosed with Alzheimer's, one comes to realize that something is terribly wrong with you. It is very frightening and then you realize, of course, that you are getting worse and that there is nothing you can do about it. There is an overwhelming dread that you soon won't be able to take care of yourself and that you will have to depend on someone to take care of you. Not at first, really, but as you move along through the diagnosis, is when you realize that you are in a situation in which there is no way out.

My first thoughts were, "I have had all of this life that is good. It is time to get out."

I thought along those lines for quite sometime. I slowly came to realize that I am still enjoying life. I do all I can and push and fight this thing as hard as I can. I was never a quitter and I am not going to start now. There are many hard things you must do in your life. The saddest thing I can think of is to give up. It takes a little courage and a little humor helps as well.

During the diagnosis, one of the Doctors asked. "How has this memory loss affected you?"

"Well, I can't do some of the things that I once did. I can't write a check anymore. I can't count without screwing up. Numbers really make me dizzy. I think that is one of the things that frighten me the most. I was always a whiz in math. I took all of the courses that I could in school because it was an easy "A". Now it is a challenge just to make change. I can't drive anywhere I want anymore, I get lost so easily. I can't find my way out of an office building or especially a hospital. All of the rooms and corridors look alike to me. It is spooky and frightens me." I said.

"So what do you do when something happens?" the doctors ask.

"So far I just drive around until I see something familiar and get my bearings from there. If I get lost in a hospital or somewhere like that, I have always found someone that will help. Guardian Angels, I call them. I don't worry much about it anymore."

The thing that does worry me most is when "time" seems to disappear. I can be driving down the road, say for example, to the Arkansas place. I can remember leaving town. The next minute, I am in Alexandria, some ninety miles away. That wouldn't bother me so much but I might have the radio tuned to a Lafayette station and would have been out of range for over an hour when I happen to notice I have been listening to static for at least an hour. No one does that.

I can't help trying to decide just when this disease could have started. It is hard to pin down. It is so subtle and slow. We have all had some incident that has happened to us that would cause us to worry. One of the first things I can remember that might be cause for alarm happened early in 1986. I was on my way from Atlanta to Baton Rouge when the airplane developed some kind of trouble and had to divert to Memphis. It seemed they had better facilities there in case we had real trouble landing. The plane landed without incident and they gave us all our tickets back and said, "This plane is not going anywhere for quite sometime. If you must get to Baton Rouge tonight, get there the best way you can. There are other flights you can take tonight."

I went to a bank of telephones and called my answering service in Lafayette to check my messages and to tell them I would be delayed in Memphis for a while, just in case anyone needed to talk to me.

I noticed a pretty lady on the phone to my left was having trouble getting her call through. It seemed that her credit cards were still in her luggage and she only had small change with her at the time. She needed to get in touch with her daughter who was waiting for her at the airport in Baton Rouge. She didn't have enough money for the phone call and they would not charge to a third party phone from a pay phone. It looked to me like she was about to panic.

I handed her my phone card I was still holding in my hand and said. "Here dahlin, use this."

She thanked me and put through her call. When I finished my conversation with the answering service, I hung up and walked away, trying to find another fight to Baton Rouge. I never thought another thing about my credit card. I found another flight later that night and ended up getting home without too much delay

Two or three nights later, I was at my home watching the TV news when the phone rang. I answered. There was a lady's voice on the other end. "Larry?" she asked.

"Yes."

"This is Kathleen."

I racked my brain for a moment. "I am afraid you have the advantage." I said. I don't think I know a Kathleen."

"Yes, I met you just the other night in Memphis." she said.

"Lady, you must be putting me on. I haven't been in Memphis in years." I started to hang up, thinking it must be one of those crank calls you hear about.

"At the airport. You loaned me your credit card. Remember?" she said quickly. "I got your name and number from the card, but I don't know your address so I can send it back to you. Along with a few dollars to pay for the call, of course."

Now I remembered. "Yes, I forgot about it." I wondered if I would have ever remembered what happened to the card the next time I wanted to use it and it was not in my wallet. I gave her my address and then said, "I don't remember what you looked like. I guess I was somewhat in a hurry. don't worry about the money. It could not have been more than a couple of bucks."

"You know, I have some new photos that my daughter made me take. I'll send you one of them along with your phone card." she said. "Don't worry about not remembering about the card. We all went through quite an ordeal on the plane. It could have been catastrophic, you know!"

"I suppose, but what the hell, we are all still here and still alive." I said. We chatted for a few moments more and hung up. How could such a thing happen to me, I thought. I have never forgotten a credit card or anything like that in my life. Uncertainty was setting in.

The letter with the credit card came in a few days. In keeping with her word, she had sent a photo of herself as well. She was the most beautiful lady I had never seen in my life. How could I have forgotten seeing her at the airport in Memphis? She would have stood out in any crowd. On the back of the photo she had written her phone number. I picked up the phone and dialed her immediately.

She answered right away. We talked for a long time, finally made a dinner date for the next Friday after she got off work. We met at a restaurant. I recognized her right away. She sparkled in the light. I was proud to have her on my arm as we walked into the restaurant. I should have paid more attention to my mother when she told me when I just a little kid, "Everything that glitters is not gold."

All in all, we hit it off rather nicely. We had another date for the next Sunday for brunch in New Orleans. She always met me at a public place rather than at her home. It was only after the third date that she told me where she lived and where she worked. She worked for the FBI. I should have run, not walked, out of her life right then, but again, I couldn't help feeling a little proud when I went into a club or restaurant with that gorgeous woman hanging on my arm.

I have since figured out why people who work for the FBI, the IRS or any of the other opprobrious occupations, don't want anyone to know their occupations or where they live. It is because if the neighbors know, no one will talk to them and no one will play with their kids. The neighbors drop them like a bad habit.

We dated for about a year and a half. The first year was great. We went everywhere together. We were inseparable for that first year. I thought I had fallen forever in love. It was during the second year that things started falling apart. I could not do anything right, according to her. I ate too fast. I combed my hair wrong. I wore the wrong clothing. She thought I should always wear a coat and tie. (It was only recently that I quit wearing blue jeans and a tee shirt to the Country Club.) She even told me that I mowed the grass the wrong way. How in the hell can you mow grass the wrong way? I can recall one time a the Petroleum club when she said to me, "Larry, you are eating too fast."

"Who in the hell set the standard for how fast one eats?" I asked.

"I just read in an Army Vanderbilt book, that you should take a bite, lay your fork down, and chew your food sixteen times before swallowing," she stated.

"Well, I just finished reading a "Time and Motion" study from MIT that said eating your way was Bull shit."

She got mad. "I just tell you these things because I want you to be a better person."

"Damn it, I like the way I am, if I didn't, I would change. I have been living this way, combing my hair this way and wearing comfortable clothes for almost fifty years. Please don't try to make me over into something I am not. You know, they say that the only things a female can change about a male is his diaper. If you want a God-damned Banker, you should go find one."

"Let's drop it before I get mad," she said.

"You are always mad about something. You have never once seen me angry. You have never even heard me raise my voice. To me, it only shows ignorance. You can't be living a happy life, mad all the time."

"You don't deal with the people I do," she said in almost a whisper.

"Then you should QUIT…. Do something else." Silence.

Then" "Look darlin, if you want a nice, sweet, gentle, man, you have him. If you want a Goddamn Banker that wears a suit and tie all the time, then I had just better hit the dusty road."

About six months later she did tell me to hit the road. That it was over. Down deep inside of me, I was glad. She said that I had hurt her feelings when I didn't show up at a birthday party she was having for me. I am truly sorry about hurting anyone's feelings, and I wondered how I could have forgotten an important date so easily.

"Well darlin," I said sincerely, "You have helped me through some dark days after my wife died, and you have brightened up the rest of them. God bless you, I will never forget you."

Tears were starting to flow from her eyes. "Maybe I have been a little hasty. Maybe we should give it one more try?"

"I think not," I said. "It would just be something else later on. We have a lot of good memories, let's just leave it like that."

"Boy, we do have the memories. Remember that time when we were coming back from Cancun and we missed the last plane to Baton Rouge and you had to rent a car in Houston? Remember how we got stopped for speeding in some little town and you convinced that cop that you were driving an FBI agent to Baton Rouge and that you had diplomatic immunity?"

"Well, it didn't hurt to try, and the ID of yours didn't hurt either. It looked like a menu from some fancy restaurant. He looked like one of those cops that you see in a B movie, didn't he? The kind that has lines like, "You're in a heap of trouble boy. My brother-in-law is the judge and he don't cotton to no Damn Yankee comin down here and hauling ass through his county."

She laughed then. "You always were the fastest thinker I ever saw. Larry…I am going to miss all of that, one thing you certainly taught me is how to live. You could work a hundred hours in a row out on an Oil Rig in the Gulf of Mexico and the next night we could be lying on a beach in Ambergris Cay on the Isla Mujeres or some other place."

"Hey, I work hard and I play hard."

She was laughing now but the tears were still there. "Remember that time in Belize when you had all of the people around us thinking that I was Loni Anderson" You must have had twenty people lined up behind you wanting to get my autograph. You were speaking to them in Spanish and I had no idea what was going on. Remember?"

"Yeah, those third world cesspools are something else, aren't they? Remember when they were landing the plane, the pilot had to make a pass over the runway to get the monkeys and other creatures off the cement so they could land the plane…. Really, that is all ancient history, baby. It is obvious to me that we are chasing different dreams. It would never work. Let's cut our losses and call it quits now, today. Let's face the facts. This had been an incongruous relationship from the beginning."

She said nothing.

"Look, I have got to get to the airport. I have got to pick up my daughter. She has been in the Bahamas for a couple of months and I am looking forward to seeing her. I don't want her to have to wait…. Again, darlin, God bless you and please know that I will never forget you. I walked out sad and happy at the same time.

She must have called me a dozen times over the next few months. I was always pleasant to her on the phone, but I never accepted any of her invitations to dinner or other such affairs. "We were happy most of the time, were we not?" she would ask.

"I think so, and then we met." I was joking, I think.

Looking back, I believe that the credit card affair and forgetting the birthday party were possibly some of the first signs of this Alzheimer's thing. I only mention and tell you a little about my affair with Kathleen because it was the memory loss that was instrumental in meeting her. I would never have met her had I just remembered to pick up the phone card when she was finished and of course, it as forgetting about the birthday party that caused me to lose her. Part of going through life, I suppose.

6

Stages

The doctors tell me (this is a direct quote) "In the First Stage, the disease begins very gradually, often with minor symptoms, perhaps some mood changes. No one notices anything wrong. The person seems to have less energy, less drive, less spontaneity, is slower to learn anything, forgets some words, (most often nouns) is slower to react, avoids anything new and often seeks out things that are familiar."

Looking back, I seemed to fit that mold exactly. The experts say there are five separate stages of Alzheimer's disease. We will address each in later chapters. By the way, don't look for a happy ending to this book or you will be disappointed. I have stated before that I believe this illness is caused by fate. Now I don't know. Fate may have caused the disease, but I think each of us is driven by something else. An incurable disease devastates some; others don't let it bother them at all. I fall somewhere in-between.

Let me say that forgetfulness is not necessarily one of the early signs of Alzheimer's Realizing that you have forgotten something may only be a sign that you are simply aging normally. The Alzheimer's patient is aware that something is wrong, but doesn't quite know what it is and is likely to act as if nothing is wrong. You get good at covering up. You get fantastic at covering up. I can change the subject quicker than anyone you know.

I would say the first thing to look for is mood change, confusion and unusual irritability. Again I am speaking form my own experience. I realize that I am slowly and progressively losing mental function. The things I once did well, I now can't do at all. Most things I won't even try to do at all. One tends to avoid anything that might lead to failure.

It is important to keep a sense of humor, I think. Just a few days ago, I was hanging out at the Racquet Club, drinking Coke and talking with some friends. A lady that was a stranger to me asked if I wanted to play a set or two of tennis.

"I am sorry, no, I said. "I just can't move fast enough to play tennis anymore Old age, I suppose."

"It probably wouldn't be much of a match anyway," she said. "I turned pro when I was 16. How about Gold? I shoot in the low eighties."

"No thanks, they say I stand too close to the ball, AFTER I shoot. The only club I own anymore is a 7 iron and I just use it to kill snakes with." I stated.

A game of Pool then?" she asked.

"Haven't played pool in years. Sorry."

"Darts?"

"Sorry."

"You can't seem to do anything," she said with some sarcasm.

"I can do one thing that you can't," I stated.

"What is that? We might make it a contest."

"I can pee standing up. Want to give it a go?"

All my friends died laughing. The lady left without saying another word. "I'll bet Will Rogers never met you, did he?" I said as she was walking away. Haven't seem her since. Takes all kinds of people to make a world.

Someone said, "Don't worry about her, Larry. She is one of the snowbirds that are only here for the winter. She will be going back north soon."

To continue: When the loss of skills, mood swings and confusion become too obvious to ignore, it is time to see the doctor. If you are not as lucky as I to have a dear friend who is a doctor and a very good one, I might add, seek out the very best one you can find. You are going to need an advocate if the ultimate diagnosis is indeed Alzheimer's. You won't be going to just one. Alzheimer's lacks a Biological marker. Whereas most other diseases are easily identifiable with certain bacteria, etc., With Alzheimer's, your doctors must be medical detectives. I think, with me, and I am sure with most, they use what is called "Diagnosis by Exclusion."

In looking through the reams of paper from am multitude of doctors, I have weeded out some of the things they looked for in me. An MRI to search for a brain tumor or a blood clot, as well as evidence of a series of small strokes they call "Multiinfarct Dementia."

They asked about over medication...I wasn't taking any medication at all. Next was an Ultra-Sound to determine if any of the blood vessels were clogged, limiting the blood flow to the brain. I had about 30% blockage in one artery. Not alarming, they said.

Alcoholism, drug abuse, malnutrition, vitamin deficiencies, the Endocrine system and metabolic disorders can all produce symptoms that closely resemble Alzheimer's

They even tried treating me for a couple of months for Depression, which can be mistaken for Alzheimer's'. They gave me antidepressant drugs. Didn't help.

There are many other incurable mental disorders that are akin to Alzheimer's. Picks, Parkinson's, Huntington's, and something called Cruetfields Jakob as well as the rare Kuru. Some respond to medication for a while. With others the prognosis is the same as Alzheimer's.

You will also need a thorough physical exam. They take blood, stool samples, etc., and an electrocardiogram every time you turn around, it seems.

Given the multitude of possible diagnosis, you can see how difficult it is to put all of the pieces together to get a definite diagnosis of Alzheimer's. My advice would be, again, to seek out the very best that you can find and afford, if you don't have a family doctor, I would go to your local medical society or a teaching hospital. There is one in almost every major city. The National Institute on Aging has a number of centers in the United States. They may be able to refer you to a good doctor, or better yet, The Alzheimer's Association.

Get a friend that knows you well to help you with a complete medical history. To the doctors, this is most important. Write everything you and your friends and family can think of on the subject. From hobbies to diet. Leave out nothing. It is all-important. If it is a silly statement, they will skip over it. It may seem silly to you, but not to your doctor.

Sooner or later in your diagnosis, you are going to be sent to a psychiatrist. He (or She) will spend some time looking for signs of an emotional upset that can be treated, such as, the death of a spouse or child, (God Forbid,) the loss of your job or family conflicts and the like. Expect these questions.

Then you will be asked questions like: Where is this place? What is this place? What town is this? What is the date? Who were the least three (or four) Presidents? These are all standard questions. Other exams include putting pegs in holes, aligning colored blocks into a certain pattern and such. I can't remember many more right now, but I know I have spent hours and hours going through all these tests that can best be termed "Child's Games".

You will be stuck with pins, tapped with a rubber hammer and any number of other things. All designed to determine the presence of a treatable condition or in the alternative, ALZHEIMER'S. These tests are not cheap, but as I stated before, seek out the best you can afford, you will need your advocates when you apply for your disability insurance or Social Security Disability. The more "World Renowned" doctors you have, the better, it seems.

Alzheimer's is expensive. Only the very rich or the very poor (on some sort of Government medical program) can afford it. It will break the middle class. I couldn't tell you how many tens of thousands of dollars I have spent so far and it is still going on.

I have told you of the first stages as they were told to me. The second stage is a follows: The person can still perform familiar activities, but may need help with more complicated things Understanding is much slower. Speech is much slower. You find it hard to make decisions or you may make unwise ones. You become more insensitive to the feelings of others. AND, PLEASE, don't take this personal; it is only out of frustration and confusion. Further, your patient will avoid situation that may lead to failure, whether it is making a home repair or Sex.

Understand that these symptoms of the Five Stages I am telling you about are not my thoughts. They were compiled from all the doctors I have seen through the past three or four years. However, I agree with them, as I am sure you will.

Just because you exhibit some or all of the symptoms I have just described above does not necessarily mean that you have Alzheimer's but you should start thinking about seeing your doctor. It could be nothing but stress, vitamin deficiency, any number of things. Even if the diagnosis turns out to be Alzheimer's, it need not be all doom and gloom. It does not mean that the person cannot still function very well in society. There are prototype treatments and the sooner you get started on one, the better.

Third Stage: It is not obvious that the person is disabled. Recent memories are very poor while memories of long ago are still sharp and vivid. The person forgets dates, times, even the season. Doesn't know where he is at times. The person may invent or substitute inappropriate words in conversation. May not recognize familiar people or even family members. Instructions must be made very clear and repeated often.

They tell me the third stage is the stage that I am in at this time. The early third. Moderate, I think is the words they use. By now you will know and everyone else will know that something is wrong. One of the first things to go for me was numbers…Math, I can't count anymore. I can't make change. No matter how hard I try, I can't learn it back. I have tried for a year, but to no avail. I know that two and two are four, but don't put it on paper and ask me to solve the problem. It is like an abstract drawing, it makes no sense at all.

It is not exactly true that I don't understand the number four. When someone says four, I can visualize four things—four fingers, bananas, etc. Ten to the Tenth power, I don't understand. It has no meaning at all. Quadratic equations, prime numbers, square root, Inverse Square are all things I once used in my engineering work but now have NO meaning. I recently read somewhere that some mathematician has discovered the largest prime number that has been discovered to date. It is 2 to the 132,049^th power, minus 1. I suppose it may be nice to know for conversation down at the pool hall but I can't imagine any mathematician spending their time trying to find a prime number that high. May be there is a use for it, but what? It would take longer than the age of the Universe to calculate and of course the number would be higher than the number of atoms in the Universe. I would rather they would tell me now many gallons of gas it would take me to get to Little Rock.

When I was a kid. I took all of the math classes in school that they offered. It was an easy "A." I always thought Math was a certainty. That Math would be the one thing that would be free from paradox and contradiction. As I grew older, I learned that the foundation of that certainty is cracking. There will always be paradoxes, questions that math will never solve, i.e. the axiom of set theory.

I relate the finding of a cure for Alzheimer's disease to the Continuum Hypotheses. No Mathematician has ever proven it true or false. There is a thirds status. It is undecidable. It cannot be proved or disproved based on present day axioms. I think that means that the present day axioms of set theory doesn't tell us enough about sets to decide the questions.

A French Mathematician, I forget his name, spent all his life trying to prove the continuum theory. All his theories proved wrong, of course, does that mean the someone should not go no trying? I think not. It would help if one knew before hand that such theories could or could not be proven.

Conversely, does that mean that just because scientists have not found a cure for Alzheimer's, they should not go on trying? Another paradox, in my view. Some scientists say that under a certain set theory, it can't be done. Other scientists say that under another Certan set theory, it can. They just can't decide which. With the knowledge about the cause of Alzheimer's that is known today, there is not enough information for medical science to get a complete picture. It is my understanding, that the cause of the disease poses some questions. Some say that it could be heredity others say environment or toxic poison. I have also heard that is may be a slow virus. A real cause may never be known or there may be dozens of causes.

I read in the Arkansas Democrat newspaper recently where a team of international researchers led by Dr. Sue Griffin of the Central Arkansas Veteran's Healthcare System released findings that bring a cure one step closer to reality. Dr. Griffin's team found that those who inherit the gene IL-1A2 and IL-1B2, from both parents have a much higher chance of developing Alzheimer's. The findings reveal the gene encodes a protein call Interleukin-1 that helps the brain's neurons heal after an injury or the normal wear of aging. The production of

Interleukin-1 normally ceases when the repair is complete. However in the inherited gene brain, Interleukin-1 is produced beyond the repair, leading to the forming of plaque in the brain. As the plaque expands, it damages the brain further and the cycle continues. It will ultimately interfere with normal brain activity and lead to the symptoms of Alzheimer's. Could it be that this gene might be the marker that the research people have been searching for all these years? These findings are encouraging because it may lead to an earlier detection and treatment. Some doctors believe even at this date that some medications can temporarily reduce memory problems and delay the onset of symptoms.

Griffin goes on to explain why anti-inflammatory drugs, such as Ibuprofen, appear to slow the onset of Alzheimer's symptoms. The pill decreases the production of Interleukin-1, which drives the body's attack against foreign proteins after injury. Researchers can now develop remedies that target Interleuykin-1 in the brain, but not will reduce its effect throughout the body.

Another Giant Step, BUT, is this just a treatment for a type of Alzheimer's that may be caused from brain injury? The data is too fragmentary to draw a scientific conclusion at this time.

What can each of us patients do to help solve this Paradox? I have always been a positive and energetic man. I volunteer for any research project that comes along. These include drug studies for experimental drugs. Letting the students at the University give me their battery of mental status tests. They are trying to compile a set of questions that will help in the diagnosis. All of these things will be of some value in time. Even if it just proves to be of no value, it will provide them some information that they are on the wrong track.

I would highly suggest any Alzheimer's patient do the same. What have you go to lose? And maybe, just maybe, you will be the first person to be cured from this nefarious disease. Wouldn't that be something to be written about in the medical journals?

7

Drug Studies

As I stated in an earlier narrative, I have been involved in a drug study program for the past two or three years. Although it is over now, I was one of the ones that did well on the drug. I was told there were two of us that went from a base line, (on the mental status test) of fifteen to twenty-one. I don't have any idea what that means except to say that having twenty-one of anything is better than having only fifteen. Hair, teeth, dollars, anything, with the possible exception of Bill Collectors. The drug manufacturer however is not going to continue that particular drug because the rest of the study group didn't do so well. They either stayed the same or declined. There were not enough positive results to continue the study to the point of FDA approval.

To continue, don't press for a diagnosis. Most of your really good doctors are very conscientious and will approach a diagnosis with caution. Especially in a case of suspected Alzheimer's. If they finally tell you, or in some cases, your family members, that it is Alzheimer's', there is no need seeking further tests. The chances are good that they are right. Spend your remaining energies adjusting to the situation. Be happy that you have the advantage of an early diagnosis and have the time to plan for the future, take that dream vacation, take up golf or other long postponed pleasures.

Don't spend a lot of time looking for that miracle cure. There are none. There are a lot of things you can do to help the situation though. The Doctors have me taking a lot of the "B" vitamins; B-12, a B complex, Folic acid and the E vitamin. I recently read that researchers at the Institute of Psychiatry and Maudsly Hospital in London found that 60% of their Alzheimer's patients were deficient in vitamin E. Review has pointed out areas of possible flaws in that study. I heard that Lecithin was also a boon. I ate that damn stuff by the spoonful, to no avail. Further, there are certain foods to avoid but I can't give you a list. Best ask for your doctor for his advice on diet.

I recently heard that Nicotine could be helpful in delaying the progression of Alzheimer's. They are doing a study right now in Japan and in Australia and they have found Nicotine to be of some value in delaying the progression of Alzheimer's. Try telling that to some of the "in your face" militant, non-smokers. Really, they are even prescribing nicotine patches for those who do not smoke. Might be worth a try. What the hell, if you are going to die anyway, it might as well be from lung cancer as Alzheimer's. The bright side is that Lung Cancer might take 30 or 40 years to kill you. Hell, you will probably be dead by that time anyway. They do say that no heavy smoker has ever died from Alzheimer's. True? I don't know. I wouldn't know how to research that concept.

So now what? You have done your homework on what you should do. You go to the Library to find out exactly what this strange disease is all about. You won't find much that is helpful. I asked the librarian if the two or three books of Alzheimer's were all that they had. Her statement to me was that we didn't need any more books on Alzheimer's. That everything that can be said about the disease has already been said. What a stupid statement. Stupidity never ceases to amaze me. Maybe we should close the United States Patent Office because everything that is worthwhile has already been invented.

I went to a bookstore, not far from where I live. The woman behind the counter asked if she could help me find something.

"Yes, maybe you can. I am looking for some books on Alzheimer's disease." I stated.

"Oh no. We won't handle any books like that at all," she said with some disgust.

"Really, why not?" I asked.

"Well, the owner of this store is really religious," she said.

"So am I. What in hell has religion got to do with it?"

"Alzheimer's is the work of the devil," she stated flatly.

"I'll be damned. That is sure good to know. All I need is an exorcist." Just when I think I have heard everything, some idiot makes a statement like that...Get used to it.

The diagnosis will be a shock to everyone and you will need time to absorb that bad news. I would say it is tantamount to a doctor telling you that you have incurable Cancer and you have very little time left. Schedule an appointment with a specially trained social worker in a week or two, after you have had time to settle down a little. They can tell you about the helpful resources that are available to you and your family.

Above all, immediately get in touch with the Alzheimer's association and ask for all the literature they have avail-able. They will be of tremendous help. They will recommend ways and things that can be done to improve the quality of life for the patient and the caregiver as well.

You may be able to cope with this disease in the beginning without much assistance, but it is important to get your ducks in a row for the future.

You will be devastated at first. You can think of all sorts of ways to end it all. DON'T DO IT! Those thoughts will soon be gone and you may be able to go on for many years, having all kinds of fun and doing the things that you never took the time to do before. I have said it before and it seems I can't say it enough.

The woods and mountains are my respite. You can learn a new appreciation for nature while you are watching a deer feed on wild pears or my old neighbor's corn. Perhaps a squirrel building a nest in an old white oak tree or a hundred other things that nature provides. Humming birds fascinate me. I can watch them for hours as they fight over their spot at the feeders I have hanging on the porch. Little things like that can take away your stress and put you more at ease with your plight.

8

Are Your Affairs in Order?

Assuming that you are lucky enough to have gotten an early diagnosis, you will have time to get your legal things in order. I would first make a list of your assets. Have someone help you with this. Make yourself a checklist. Include such things as:

Social Security Number. Your Lawyer. Your Will, if you don't have one, make one. You must do this while you are still mentally alert. It would be advisable to move as quickly as you can on this matter.

List all of your insurance policies, safety deposit boxes, stock certificates, and personal property, (especially real estate), credit cards, outstanding loans, including money owed to you etc. Although it didn't do me a hell of a lot of good, as you know, if you read my first book. Don't forget to label your keys. Keys to every lock you own. House, car, safety deposit boxes, the gate, anything. Get a label put on them.

I don't have a will. I have a limited partnership and several trusts. That way there is no probate or no succession for your kids to go through. All they have to do is elect another General Partner and continue the business or sell out, whatever they decide. I might mention those Limited Partnerships and trusts are very complex and can be very expensive to set up. You must have a lawyer to do this for you as well as a good accountant to look after your taxes and the like. But, they can save your family a lot of headaches later. I don't want my heirs to have to go through the court system to take control of my property when I die. I just don't trust our Legal system or in my view, you can call it an Illegal system. I have never met a *GOOD* Judge. I am not saying there aren't any, just that I have never met one. *Justice is an abstract; completely devoid of reality!*

Find someone you can trust and give the power of attorney. Someone to handle all of your affairs for you. They should keep detailed records of all your financial affairs. Find someone that you would trust with your life.

If you don't have a lawyer, your local bar association should be able to help you find one. Also, the Legal counsel for the Elderly in Washington, D. C. can help. Write or call them. They can recommend someone in your area.

Health insurance can be another problem. If you don't have insurance, you probably won't be able to get any. I have tried several companies about supplemental insurance. They won't even talk to me. The best I could do was buy a policy through AARP that pays a flat amount for every day you are in a Hospital, for whatever reason. You can get fifty dollars a day or a hundred, two hundred, just any amount you can afford. It is not much but it is better than nothing. Those kinds of policies are not usually very expensive.

I hear that several major insurance companies are soon going to be offering a new policy covering long term care. It might be worth checking into that possibility. Medicare is only partial protection, as you may know. Check your Social Security office for updated brochures. Most of the needs of the Alzheimer's patient will not be covered by Medicare and if you are lucky enough to find a "Medigap" insurance that you can afford, you will find that it has its limitation as well. At any rate, insurance is not something you should buy impulsively.

Nothing you can do will ever make you "Ready" for this disease. The enormous demands, the changes that you will be going through every day, are the hardest work you will ever do in your life. Even more so than losing that extra twenty or thirty pounds that have put on over the past few years.

Keep in mind that the Changes that are happening to you not only affect you, but everyone around you. Your caregiver may need special help and support. If you are a caregiver, find a support group in your area. If there are none, start one. I know that finding just one other person in the same situation will help you beyond anything else you can do. For me, just finding one other Alzheimer's patient that was just like me was the best thing that could have happened to me, my friend, Diana. We talk or write or E-mail each other constantly. We help each other out with the sadness that patient and caregivers alike are going to have from time to time. Remember that the more calm and cheerful a caregiver can be will be a boon to the patient. I know that a hug or a pat on the shoulder can have calm, soothing results. We patients can be very intuitive. We can sense in a second when something is wrong. We like things running smoothly. AND, PLEASE, don't assume that we are going to act like normal people. Sometimes our antenna is pointed at another station. We are marching to the beat of a different drummer. The reasons of which are shrouded in this mysterious disease.

If you are close to an Alzheimer's patient, there may be times when your feelings are hurt by a sudden aloofness. This is a reaction to a situation and probably not directed at you personally. Please, please, don't take these things personal. It may just be that his mind is wandering or the apparent withdrawal is merely to clear his head and see things more clearly from a distance. If a mistake is made, don't act as if it were unforgivable. A warm smile, a hug, or a pat on the back can work wonders. An AD Patient is susceptible to a touch when it is gentle. Anything else is a definite turn-off.

Speaking for myself, I rely on my emotions. I can quickly spot a fraud and can respond instinctively to the sincerity in others. Don't make the mistake of underestimating the intelligence of an AD patient. It is there but doesn't display itself in social repartee. No matter how much evidence there is to the contrary, this stereotype holds. It seems folks still talk to us like we just fell off the turnip truck.

It is not easy to find information on Alzheimer's. The kind you may be seeking. If you are like me, I wanted to find something of what to expect, what other patients were going through, etc. Until recently, Alzheimer's was not a well-publicized disease. I have found that most people don't know anything about it. I have begun to hear more and more about it on the radio and on TV. We are all starting to get more knowledgeable about this disease. Just today I heard Dr. Dean O'dell saying that for a girl born this year, her chances of contracting Alzheimer's during her lifetime is one in six. For a male the chances are one in nineteen. Something to think about. There were more statistics but I couldn't write them down fast enough and I forgot them. With near four million patients in the Untied State alone and the fourth-leading cause of death among older Americans, don't assume that you can't be afflicted. Do Something There are three kinds of people in the word, I am told. Those that make things happen, those that watch things happen, and those that wonder what happened.

Where to start. You might try seeking out a primary caregiver. Give him or her a respite. Get involved. Learn about the disease. Learn about the little quirks of the patient. Be the friend you can be. Volunteer some of your time at a nursing home that takes care of AD patients. Read to them, feed them, shave them, whatever you can do. Use your imagination. Anything will help. Anything to boost the morale and demands of the disease. I remember someone asking Mother Teresa what someone that had little money or resources could do to help make a better world. Her answer? Smile a lot."

I know from experience that a smile and a few kind words can make all the difference. I recall once several years ago when I was still working, I stopped into the café about two in the morning to get some coffee. The little waitress was from China. She was a student over at the University. She had been serving some teenagers over in a booth. When she came to the counter where I sat, she was crying.

"What's wrong, Darling?" I asked.

"Those guys in the booth said that my eyes looked funny. They wanted someone else to wait on them," she replied through the tears.

"Don't pay any attention to a bunch of illiterates like that, sweetie. It is obvious they don't know real beauty when they see it. They wouldn't know a Ming Dynasty Vase from a can of Beer." The smile I got from her made me feel good for a week.

"You're special," she said.

Those words made me feel even better…. And it didn't cost a dime.

I must be hard to understand at times. People are continually asking me to repeat. If I listen to myself talk, I find myself using words in an idiom once totally foreign to me. Locutions like "It's not hook up," or "Ain't so." There was a time when I was very precise in my grammar; a time when I would never use such an illiteracy.

It seems that I can still write though. The words come through my fingers when I can't use the same words orally. I usually know what I want to say but the words get stuck somewhere. Other times I will use a wrong word or say something totally inappropriately, like if someone asks how I am feeling today, I might catch myself saying "Ball" or changing the subject by saying something like, "There is a cat in the parking lot." Another paradox?…. Perhaps.

9

A Few Kind Words

I have told you so much about the derogatory things some people say to me from time to time. It is those times when I would like to remember every little slight and when I get a chance, to drop a Safe on their head. That soon passes. Other times people can he so understanding and will go out of their way to make me feel good. Such a thing happened to me just a day or so ago.

I was coming out of the Post Office down in the Oil Center. Someone behind me said, "Hey Larry."

I turned around to see a total stranger. I must have had a blank look on my face. He said immediately, "Larry, I'm Sam, Sam Bennett."

I recognized the name at once, but Sam didn't look like the Sam I knew. "Oh, Hi there Sam. It's good to see you. It took me a moment…"

"I know Larry, I heard that you had been sick. I'm sorry." Sam said.

"Luck of the draw, Sam." Sam is the President and CEO of a large independent Oil Company based in South Louisiana and was a good client of mine for many, many years.

"That's one way to look at it, Larry, but it is still hard to see such a thing happen to someone like you." Sam said sadly.

"It's not doom and gloom, Sam, I am still able to get out and around a little and it is always great to see an old friend like you," I said. "I just forget things…."

"Larry, you could forget half and still be smarter than most people I know," Sam said with a smile.

"Sam, that is a real good statement and I would like to believe that it is true, but I don't…."

"Well, I do," Sam said. "Why do you think I used you and your company to do all of my wireline work in the years that I have know you?"

"Sam. What you said might not be true, but I'm glad you said it anyway. I should be getting home now. Thanks, Sam, for being my friend and give my best to your wife."

"I will sure do that, Larry, and good luck to you," said Sam.

Isn't it great how the words and a smile from someone can make a person feel good for a long time?

In my beloved Ozarks, if not in my home in Louisiana, my repertoire of friends and supporters are growing. What a mystery to me, friendships, and how diverse one's friends can be. From a Governor in a southern state to a questionable used car dealer in Texas, from a Doctor in Iran to a ginseng farmer in Arkansas. I could go on and on. They accept my condition. They accept everything about me. They are proud to be called on and they respond generously to anything asked of them and never expect anything in return. I will never understand exactly why, given my capricious personality of late. Was it just chance that brought us together? Was it divine guidance? It seems that they believe in you from the first "Hello" and never require an explanation for what can best be termed "strange behavior."

The people that live near my mountain retreat are all a; good deal like this. One morning as I was leaving the cabin to go back to Louisiana, I dropped by the Racquet Club to have coffee with the gang there. A lot of my friends were already there when I arrived. There was Sue, the activities director for the Club, Frank, Chuck and Chicago Bob and the rest. Not there that morning to my disappointment, were Dathine and Lila. Two people that had become more than just friends. More like old war buddies. I love talking to each of them.

Dathine is one of those rare women that are hard to describe. You can say that she has a trimness of a woman much younger. A mind that is tingling with life and the strength of a woman athlete. It may also be said that she has a pretty face that has seem both hard times and good, grief and joy. Her dark hair, showing a touch of gray here and there, is always neat. It would be the same if she were home alone, not expecting to see anyone. Her eyes always look square at you with a look of good comradeship and with a gleam that, to me, reveals the depth of the soul within. I am proud that she is my friend.

Lila is also a very loving person. Always, always greets you with a smile; has the body of someone much less mature and would be hard to imagine sitting in a rocking chair in front of a fire, old and withered. It wouldn't be her nature. She is so full of humor and wit that one can assume that it is her normal way. She has the ability to ask a question and before I can fully answer, with the quickness of her mind will give me a nod or a smile to show that she has caught the purpose of my reply. It is as though she has much knowledge in her mind is asleep and needs only a nudge to arouse that knowledge to life. A remarkable woman.

It is a poor picture that I paint of these friends of mine for they are all so much more than all of this I have written.

Sue, a charming woman as well as an excellent hostess, brought my coffee and joined in the conversation. I was telling the group that I had just received word from New Orleans that I had been accepted in a new drug study for an experimental drug for Alzheimer's patients. I felt that I had just won a lottery, as there were by some estimation, over four million Alzheimer's patients in the United States alone and only four hundred had been picked to participate in the new study. I was one of the four hundred. We all chatted for a time about everything from Golf to Clinton. After an hour or so, I decided to go call on my friend Lila. She did not live too far away. Seeing Dathine this trip was out of the question. She had gone to California to visit her ailing mother.

I drove away without any trouble getting out of the parking lot. I found Lila's shop right away. I startled her when I walked in. She hadn't heard me drive up. She was busy painting an oil painting of Floyd. She had told me earlier that she was going to do that for me. Lila is a world-class painter. She won first place in Arkansas last year with one of her paintings. She is so proud. We talked about the painting for a bit, choosing colors for the background etc. She then asked me. "Did you ever see all of my humming birds?"

"I haven't, Lila. Other than seeing you, that is one of the reasons I came by today."

We walked to the trees in front of her house where she had 4 or 5 bird feeders hanging from the limbs. Her house is next door to her shop. There must have been a couple of hundred of them. I had never seen anything like it in my life. She said it took about 10 pounds of sugar each week to keep them fed.

"I have only about 4 of those little birds at the cabin, Lila, and they fight like cats and dogs all the time. When one starts to eat, two more will come and chase him away."

We watched them for a while longer and then I told her I had to go. "It takes me a while to get ready to go, Lila. I must check everything over and over again before I leave, to make sure I have not forgotten anything."

She followed me to the truck. "Larry, I want you to know that Dathine and I have our whole congregation at church praying for you," she said in the most sincere voice that I had ever heard her use.

"I am so flattered that you think of me, Lila. I don't underestimate the power of prayer. You guys do so much for me. With all of you good people praying for me, how can God turn his face away?" Then: "If everyone was like you people here in the hills, this world would be a Shangri-La indeed."

"It is not all one-sided, Larry. You do so much for all of us too. You give way more than you take. It is a pleasure having you for a friend," she said with a smile and a tear.

I didn't know how to answer.

"You brighten up these hills, Larry. It is not the same when you re not here. You always have a smile and a cheerful "Hello" for everyone. You have a way of making us feel good about ourselves. You have a magnetism that I can't describe. Go ahead and go to your Doctor's appointment, but hurry back to us."

Again, I was at a loss for words. If I could have talked, I don't know what I would have said. Had it not been for this strange disease that I have, I doubt that I would have ever met these people. I would have still been in the Rat race, chasing the dollar. I drove back to the cabin, hardly knowing how I got there. I was thinking about what Lila had just told, the miles just passed away.

I took a walk down to the waterfall. I understand why our Master, Jesus, spent so much time in the wilderness, near the temples of mountains and trees that his father made. The last bars of Gold from the sun were shining through the trees onto the ground as I walked back up the trail to the cabin. The blue mist along the ridge was beginning to turn into a deeper purple. Night would be coming soon and the stars would soon be out. As I sat in the doorway of the cabin, smoking my pipe, my thoughts drifted to a quote from Shakespeare, "Not in the stars, but in ourselves, lies our destiny."

My thoughts were interrupted by the telephone. I ran to answer, thinking it might be Stella. It was not. A man asked, "Is this Larry Rose?"

"Yep." I answered.

"Congratulations, Mr. Rose. This is (So and So) from (XYZ) Sweepstakes committee and it is my pleasure to inform you that you have been selected the Grand Prize winner of a new Cadillac El Dorado."

Knowing that I had not entered a sweepstakes, I answered him, "Gee man, that's just great. I'll tell you what, just park it out in the yard with the rest of them."

"Well, Mr. Rose, we can't deliver the car to you until the sales tax has been paid. (Something like $2000.00). If you could just send us a check for that amount or if you have a credit card…"

"I don't think so," I broke in. "If I won the damn thing, just park it out in the drive way. If I didn't, we can talk about the weather. He hung up. I guess this means that I won't be getting my new Cadillac. But, I will be keeping my 2,000 bucks.

I immediately called Stella to tell her about what had just happened. She about died laughing. You did the right thing, Larry." I told her that I would be heading back to Louisiana in the morning. We chitchatted a bit more then I went to bed.

Early the next morning when I awoke, the sun was just coming over the ridge in the east. A long thin rope of mist hung in the hollow below the cabin. The sun on the clouds above turned them a bright red, tapering off to white on the western edges. I walked outside thinking that God must be very close right now.

I lifted my eyes to the red clouds above. "Hi God," I said aloud. "I've been meaning to talk to you. I thought you might help me with a couple of things. I am not going to ask to have an easy life. I would never do that. I would just ask that I be allowed to live the rest of my life free from those that do not understand me and that you might help me to spend as much time in this Beautiful place as possible."…. Then: "Aw, listen to me, God, going on about what I want. If you didn't know me so well, you would think that I didn't appreciate all of these great people that you sent to help me; and for all the other great things you have done for me in my lifetime. I know you will bless each and very one of them and keep them safe from harm. I guess I was just thinking of myself again. I know that you will do what is best for me. I'll be talking to you again later God, and thanks for everything." Was I being too pious? I thought, No,…one can't be too pious.

10

A Night Out

Back in Louisiana, I try to count down the days until the appointment in New Orleans when I will get started on the new drug. It turned out to e pretty much the same as the first one. I went through a multitude of tests, both mental and physical. I scored somewhere in the mid-range of their test requirements and was accepted. I still hate the mental status tests worst of all. They make me realize just how stupid I have become. They tell me not to worry, that I "do just fine" and that it is a very important part or the study or they would not ask me to do it again. So grudgingly, I go through it. The new medication is taken three times a day rather than the old study where I took it only two times daily. No problems so far. It is just one more thing to remember.

In a few days, my old friend, Aaron Dodge, called to ask if he, his sons and one of their friends, would go to the cabin on the next coming weekend. He wanted me to go along as well. "Sure, Aaron. You don't even need to ask. You and the boys are welcome anytime. We all went there the following weekend. I took my truck because I wanted to stay longer than just a couple of days.

IT is always good to have those kids visiting the cabin. There is never a dull moment when they are around. They always have something going on. They like to sleep in the loft and each morning when they wake up, they go out on the balcony and have what can best be described as a "pee for distance" contest. Then they cook breakfast and go down to the creek for a swim. They are blue when they get back because the water in the creek is so cold. It doesn't seem to bother the kids much though. They would rather rough it than use the shower in the cabin. They would even rather cook outside when they can. Boy Scout stuff. They are always doing something. If they are not hiking in the hills, they are fooling around with the tractor or rewiring the speakers on the stereo system. They have a hook up now for outside speakers.

In the afternoons, we would all go over to the Country Club where the boys go swimming and Aaron and I sit at one of the tables nearby and drink a coke and watch the boys and the other people. I have introduced Arson to all of my friends there. Now they are his friends as well. We love them all.

All too soon they had to leave for home. They thanked me for a great time. It was my pleasure. "Let's do it again real soon," they said.

I spent the next few days fooling around the cabin. Touching up the paint, polishing and cleaning up a little. Bonnie would come over almost every day. He kept me well supplied with tomatoes and other things from his garden. The kids love Bonnie, by the way. Such men as Bonnie are seldom seen. He is indeed something new to the boys.

One never sees Bonnie out walking the woods anymore without his gun. He was walking back down the trail to his cabin from my place one night not long ago. Somewhere along the trail, something growled at him. It scared Bonnie, so he will not go out much without a gun. A neighbor, that lives down the road a couple of miles, told me that it might have been a mountain lion. There is getting to be a lot of them around the area now.

One Friday morning, Karen from the Racquet Club, called to tell me that everyone was getting together that night around seven and that if I would like to come over and didn't feel like driving, she would send someone to pick me up and take me home when I was ready to go. How nice, I thought. I told her that I would like to come and that I could make it on my own. I have a phone in the truck and if I get screwed up, there are a couple of people I can call to help me. There is only one road to the club and if I watch carefully for the turnoff, I shouldn't have any trouble.

Karen is the new activities director over at the club, Sue, whom I mentioned earlier, is taking a long vacation with a friend. I haven't heard when she is coming back. Karen is easy to describe. One could say she is tall; beautifully tall with the trimness of a teen-age girl She is that, sort of shy, but lovely, sweet young lady that is so cheerful and full of life that anyone meeting her for the first time would know that her actions are her normal way. She is the lady dressed in white and has that image of loveliness that every man carries in a secret locket buried somewhere deep in his mind. The person that loses her for a friend would always be plagued with a vagrant, haunting memory.

I arrived at the club a little before seven with no problems. I took a little nap in the afternoon so I was refreshed and feeling good. I ordered a Club Soda at the bar, then sat at one of the tables near the dance floor. In a few minutes, everyone started filtering in.

Dathine saw me sitting alone at the table and came over to say hello. She had just returned from visiting her mother in California a day or two before. "I was hoping I would see you her tonight, Larry. I want you to sign my book for me." She had a copy of my book, "Show Me The Way To Go Home" that had just been released.

"Sure I would be glad to sign it for you," I said. I wrote in her book and handed it back to her. She read what I had written and closed the book, smiling.

"You know I have been wanting to talk to you," she said. There was a sudden solemnity in her manner as awesome as her sincerity as her head came forward over the table with a determination of conviction in what she was about to say. There are thousands of people out there who will never get to meet you, Larry, never even know that you exist, and will never know what you are going through with this damn Alzheimer's disease. Especially in the testing of these new medications," she paused for a second. Then; "And yet, whether this medicine is successful or not, will be in your debt for as long as they live. I am talking about the Alzheimer's patients throughout the world and the patients that are yet to come. You are sitting on the cutting edge of research and I know it is not a pleasant place to be. I have worked in a pharmacy, and I know the risks involved in almost any mediation, especially an experimental one."

I looked away from her. Such rhetoric is embarrassing tome. I wished something would happen that would change the subject. Do you know that if it shows this Christmas, it will be the first time in 15 years?" I made a stab at changing the subject with this ignominious statement.

"Please be serious for a moment, Larry." There is never a censorious tone in her voice. "These people I am talking about are the Alzheimer's patients that you care about, the ones you write about, try to speak for, to help," she said with her usual smile. "I know how much you care about them…I know."

"Okay, let's be serious, but let's also be honest about this. I am participating in this drug study primarily for myself. The ass that I am trying to save is mine. It would be nice to say that I am going through all of this for the good of humanity, but it wouldn't be so. When I take that pill, I am hoping and praying that it will help ME. It would be great if this drug turns out to be the magic bullet that kills Alzheimer's and that I was one of the patients that held the gun. Me and a hundred others just like me. That would be great." I took a drink of the Club Soda. She said nothing. Altruism is not my thing.

"I know that I can't be 'Larry Rose', the best Electrical Engineer in the world anymore, but I can strive to be 'Larry Rose', the best Alzheimer's patient in the world. That is just part and parcel of who I am. It appears God has given me this job to do and I intend to do the best that I can. Whatever it takes."

Then: "Some folks think that just because I wrote a book on the subject, that I live in some enchanted kingdom, or something. The fact is, when they turn out the lights and everyone goes home, this thing in my head is still there and will still be there when I get up in the morning. There is no pulling back for me, Dathine, no days off sick, no backing out of the darker days. It is peak performance all the way. I have decided that I can take one of two courses. **Course one**: I can take life as it comes and make the most of each moment, take the drugs, eat the right things, do everything that is possible to fight this thing. Or **Course two**: I can just lay down and die. The doctors tell me that I am barely at the beginning of this disease. I have to take Course one, don't you see? But, again, that is just me. I have to, at least until I am proven wrong. I won't give up easily. The book is not learned treatise, by the way. It is just my experience with this thing in my head." I saw the tears then. "Larry," I said to myself, when are you going to learn to shut up?"

Others were coming in by then, saying hello and congratulating me on the book. Dave came by and told me that his mother had just finished reading my book and now it was all he could do to keep her from buying a pig. "Thanks a lot," he joked.

I got a lot of comments that night. It appeared that about everyone there had read it. The comments were all good. Such as: "A book for the Universe." "I wish I had read it ten years ago." "I cried all the way through it." "I laughed all the way through it." All good to hear. I was a happy camper that night.

Karen was trying to get enough people together for the train ride along the White River. It runs from Calico Rock to Flippin and back. They say it is the best way to see the tree colors changing in the fall. Way out in the wilderness, away from the main traveled routes. I had to decline because I had to be in New Orleans on that day. I would have liked to have gone. Maybe another time.

The band had started playing and Dathine was trying to talk to me again. Talking over the loud music was proving to be impossible. "Let's go into the bar room for a while, Larry. It will be a little more quiet in there. I'll buy you a drink."

We went into the bar area and chose a couple of stools near the far end of the bar. "You know, Larry, I admire you so much."

I was starting to get that embarrassing feeling again. What do you mean?" I asked.

"One thing is the way you can talk to people. You may stutter and stammer a little from time to time, but you always manage to say exactly the right things. I don't think you talk or listen with your head; you do it from your heart. For example, that cute little blonde haired girl that came and asked you to dance a little while ago. You said no but you went on and made her feel that she was just about the most special person in the world just for asking. I don't know many people who can do that. The fact is, I don't know anyone who can do that."

An elderly lady came up to us then. She had a coy of my book. She asked if I would sign it for her.

"Sure, I would be delighted," I said.

"Make it to Carl and Elsie. We are here from Brighton, Colorado for a week's vacation. I am so pleased that we ran into you." She spelled Carl and Elsie for me. Cameras with flashes were going off all over the room to celebrate an occasion for someone. Perhaps a birthday. "I would also like to have your address, if you don't mind, so I can write to you from time to time. See how you are doing."

"I had them put it in the back of the book," I told her. She looked to make sure, thanked me, and went back to her table where her husband was waiting.

"You know, you draw a hell of crowd for a weekday," Dathine said with a laugh.

My old friend, Lila and her friend Ed, came by just then. Lila had a sack in her hand. "I brought you some things, Larry. I hope you like jelly!"

"For me, Lila? No way."

"Yes for you. I hope you like Muscadine jelly."

"You bet I do. I also really like that Muscatel wine. Isn't that the same grapes?" I asked.

"I think so," she said.

"I am going to make me some biscuits as soon as I get home and have some of this jelly with them."

"Well here is some Chili that I made for you as well. You may never eat chili again after this," she laughed.

"You are not going to burn those biscuits are you Larry?" Karen asked.

"Oh, Oh, I see you have been reading the book too Karen."

"It's right there in the first chapter," she said with a laugh.

"You guys treat me better than mama did. You all are going to spoil me, you know."

"Just want you to eat right while you are here," said Lila.

It was getting late for me. About 9:00PM. I really should be getting home now," I said.

"We can take you home if you want to stay longer," someone said. I knew that my words were getting fatuous and empty-headed. The longer I stayed there the more my friends would see me screwing up. I could feel myself slipping. I knew I had better be going home while I could still function. I remember a motherly hug from most everyone as was always inevitable. I, afterwards, had no recollection at all of going home. I know that I missed the trail to the cabin and ended up at a stop sign some 8 miles beyond. I never felt more alone in my life. Not unlike the malign despair of the losers in a war, I thought. This despair was not to last though. My next recollection was at seven the nest morning. Always a cheerful time of day for me. I showered, shaved and made my usual coffee. I bring my coffee with me from Louisiana. It is the New Orleans Blend that has Chicory. Most commercially available coffees are not suited to my palette. It was quiet on the mountain at this hour. The night creatures had long since gone away for the day. The first golden bars of sunlight were filtering through the trees across the hollow. God, how I love it here," I thought. But to mention more about how I love these woods, hills and the cabin would only be superfluous.

"This might be a good time to write what I have on my notes and tapes, I thought. "The cabin is clean; the grass does not need mowing. Things are looking good and I feel great." I don't have a word processor at the cabin, so I got out a notebook and started writing. Try writing about Alzheimer's without a spell check. Oh well, Susan Sullivan, the pub-lisher, did a great job with my first book. She not only edited and polished my rough manuscript, but made use of notes written on napkins from Mel's diner, backs of envelopes, etc. and made a book from all of that. She also provided a great quantity of what I needed: enthusiasm and support. She not only got into my head, but into my heart as well. There may be a few books written each year in which the author can claim sole responsibility. This is not going to be one of them.

Susan tells me at least once a week to write, write, and write. That she will do the spelling, grammar checks and pruning. She did a great job with the last book, making something out of a mountain of notes, rough pages and unprofessional and unrelated pieces of writings.

I will suppose that everyone that writes a book hopes that it will sell a million copies. The thing that I was not prepared for was the mountain of letters I received from the people that read my book. Although I would have liked to answer all of them, it was just impossible. I got letters from all over the world. From New Zealand, England, etc. One lady from Canada even sent Floyd a sack of Jellybeans. Almost all wanted me to send them a picture of Floyd.

11

Warning Signs

It was recently announced that research scientists have been able to produce Alzheimer's in mice that exhibit the same changes that take place in the brain of the Alzheimer's victims. If my understanding is right, it will mean that they can now develop new and more effective treatments than ever before. One researcher, Dr. Lieberberg, said he never expected to see this in his lifetime. It seems that they are making giant strides in research. Every inch of progress has been a hard fight. Help the Alzheimer's association if you can. They are working tirelessly against time to find a cure for this disease.

I am told that only one out of every five-research projects can be funded. The research talent exists but simply not enough dollars have been raised to fund even two out of the five promising projects.

Remember that Alzheimer's can strike almost anyone from middle age on. The early onset patients are especially heartbreaking. Those in their 40's and 50's. Most still have children and college expenses to cover along with sky-rocketing costs for medicine and care.

The Alzheimer's association tells us that no one is immune to this nefarious disease. Victims include the famous, the wealthy, the unknown and the poor. From President Reagan to the people next door. We have all heard of Rita Hayworth and her struggle with this disease. Other well known persons include: Otto Priminger, Norman Rockwell, and the mystery writer, Ross McDonald. This disease can cross race, gender as well as economic lines. No one is exempt.

I can't say it enough. Call the Alzheimer's association and ask to be put on their mailing list. If you have a loved one diagnosed with this disease or related disorder, they will continue to update you through newsletters on new things coming and tips for coping. You will need the reassurance it will bring you. You will soon be living with a stranger.

I just read that those who lead an intellectually challenging life, have advanced degrees and continue to keep their minds active are said to live longer than those who are less educated or have become stagnant. It has been said that such things as writing, playing games that require mental activity may protect and preserve you from dementia. This mental exercise theory is an exciting concept, but to date there is just not enough date to prove it. Says Steven DeKosky, MD, "We need further exploration of the mental exercise theory."

My view is, don't wait for scientific research to prove it for you. Get started yourself. Write letters to friends. Play solitaire, do some grade school math, count the steps around the block where you live, anything that will keep your mind active. Crossword puzzles are good, I find. I really like the 'FreeCell' game on the computer.

There are ten warning signs of Alzheimer's disease. These signs are compiled by the Alzheimer's association and are as follows:

1.   RECENT MEMORY LOSS THAT AFFECTS JOB PERFORMANCE

2.   DIFFICULTY PERFORMING FAMILIAR TASKS

3.   PROBLEMS WITH LANGUAGE

4.   DISORIENTATION OF TIME AND PLACE

5.   POOR OR WEAKER JUDGMENT

6.   PROBLEMS WITH ABSTRACT THINKING

7.   MISPLACING THINGS

8.   CHANGES IN MOOD OR BEHAVIOR

9.   PERSONALITY CHANGES

10. LOSS OF INITIATIVE

When you write or call the Alzheimer's association, ask for a coy of these warning sings. It will go into much more detail than I have. These are just some of the things to look for if you think someone is your family may be developing Alzheimer's disease.

12

Treatments and Hope

The days are long and the nights too, if you count nights. At one time, 6 hours of sleep was all I needed, but not these days. I have come to know that lassitude will cloud the mind. Sometimes it is absolutely necessary to sleep an hour or two in the afternoon in order to stay half way alert in the evening. Especially, when going out to some function. With this disease, one must maintain a constant state of vigilance.

As I stated earlier, Alzheimer's treatment now offers some hope. In an article written by Leslie Peacock for the *Arkansas Times*, she interviewed several of the foremost researchers in this area. When the reporter asked Dr. Pham H. Liem of the University of Arkansas for Medical Sciences, if Alzheimer's is not a fate worse than death. Dr. Liem replied. "You're out of date. Alzheimer's is not a disease that we cannot do anything about anymore. We can treat it now and the sooner the better."

Adding to Liem's optimism is research being done by Dr. Sue Griffin, who I mentioned earlier in the book. Dr. Griffin is a developmental neurobiologist at Arkansas Children's Hospital. Much of Griffin's research and her specialty is the developing brain, how it builds in the embryo. She has decided that a head injury in the adult brain seems to prompt that early brain modeling with cellular activity that is appropriate in the fetal brain. When looking at tissue samples from the Alzheimer's brain, Griffin further decided that it looked to her like a reaction to injury, an Immune system response.

To paraphrase Leslie's article, it appeared that Griffin is seeing a vicious circle in the brain in which neurons begin to die, triggering immune cells to start making Interleukin-1, the same chemical that the brain makes after a head injury. The interleukin-1 then triggers a reaction in the brain's chemistry that eventually kills more neurons and starts the process all over again. As I understand the article, the immune system goes wild and doesn't know when to shut down causing an overreaction that caused the process to become chronic.

If this is indeed the case, I may have inadvertently been taking a drug that quite probably delayed the onset of Alzheimer's. For the past ten years or so I have been taking a Non-steroid anti-inflammatory drug for arthritis. Duke University in North Carolina, as I understand, has decided that persons with rheumatoid arthritis, who have been treated with anti-inflammatory drugs, weren't as likely to develop Alzheimer's, as was the general public.

Further, Dr. Liem and his colleagues at the UAMS have found that in a three-year study, that women who take estrogen after menopause have significantly milder cases of Alzheimer's. Animal studies at Yale are also finding that estrogen seems to aid the growth of healthy neurons. Of course, my next thought would be, "What kind of side effect would estrogen have on the male patient?" Later research has determined that just the opposite may occur. One would have to say that research in this particular area is Nebulous.

Leslie also states in her article and found in her research, that Medical Science can't say just what causes Alz-heimer's. A gene has been identified, but not everyone with the gene develops the disease; and some people who have the disease don't have the gene. Also while Dr. Griffin, Dr. Liem and others in the field see the link in Alzheimer's and head injuries, a prominent Doctor that I know in New Orleans thinks that one of the causes may be a toxin in the environment.

In spite of the paradoxes in the research that is going on all over the world, there is a ray of light at the end of the tunnel. Nursing homes are beginning to take a new approach in delaying with dementia patients and to sustain that education, Cornelia Beck, an Associate Dean in the School of Nursing at UAMS has stated, "People have not been taken care of with a lot of understanding." Beck and her colleagues have been devising ways for caregivers to talk and to work with patients to maintain their basic living skills. I think because of her and her efforts, a lot of life and basic living skills will be sustained in patients in nursing homes. Thank you, Cornelia!

Ostensibly, the use of anti-inflammatory medication may well be a boon to the Alzheimer's patient. My dear friend and fellow patient, Diana McGowin, has been taking INDOCIN for the past couple of years. She too has been on a plateau for some time. Ask your doctor about it. At best it may help, at the worst, innocuous.

I just mentioned the word, 'Plateau'. While on a TV talk show with Dr. Richard Strub, MD, Chairman, Dept. of Neurology at the Ochsners Clinic in New Orleans, heard the mention of Plateau, either by me or someone else on the show. He stated that to him, it is a strange word in describing a stage in the disease. He stated that although the disease may seem quiescent for a time, it is degenerative and still progressing. He thinks that I am just in a stage right now where everything I am doing I can do and that I will not attempt to do anything that might lead to failure. He thinks that I may exhibit a heightened responsiveness quite alien to personality previously manifest, simply because I am on a roll right now. The book signings, the TV and Radio shows and everything that is keeping me busy right now. "When you are feeling good about yourself, you think better," Strub stated. "Not unlike when a person is depressed, with no disease, they don't think too clearly. When they get to feeling a little better, they start thinking more clearly."

When it became known on the show that I was having trouble tying my shoes and buttoning my shirt, Dr. Strub explained that it is a natural progression of Alzheimer's disease. We give it a fancy name, APRAXIA. It means a loss of skilled and purposeful motor acts. Things that once came easy are now a little more difficult. It seems to me that the Doctors have a word for everything I do. When I get a little tired, I can't do anything well at all, SUNDOWNERS, they say. When I am unable to recognize objects or people, AGNOSIA. I had never heard of these words before. I guess they have been around a long time. The words were not an archetype just for me.

I think I am doing well. I am writing on my second book. As Dr. Strub says, "I am on a roll." Stella says that I have cut myself off from most people. To her, I have reduced my basic needs to the point of just eating, sleeping, writing and listening to music. I suppose that is the way she sees it. To me, an extraordinary calm has descended over me. A feeling I have never known before. A secret microcosm that is impossible to turn away from. I am not at all sure that I want to. I am quite happy here in my little pit of mediocrity; if only I could put aside the frustration and fear of the unknown that overcomes me from time to time I am safe. I am in danger, back and forth. I can't seem to shake that feeling.

I was telling my son, Jeff, just the other day that there is so much more to life than just the quest for knowledge and wealth. Learning about kindness, courage and love are paramount. That is something that has to come from inside a person. You can't learn these things from books.

"I think the thing I will miss most about you, Dad, are the fruits of your wisdom; Jeff said, among hundreds of other things. We have been deer hunting in South Texas, Elk hunting in Colorado, the canoe trips down the Little Red, sailing to Belize on the boat and just hanging out. You always seemed to have it all together. We have just about done it all, you and me. I am going to miss that."

There was little I could say. I remained silent.

13

Talk Shows

I continue getting letters from folks all over. People from other continents, people of every color, in languages I have never read before; from countries whose borders I have never crossed. They all say about the same thing. They laugh, they cry, they can't put the book down until they have read the last page. AND they all say THANKS for sharing your life with us. Some send pictures of their families or their pets.

I don't think any; of them realize that this book was a last desperate chance to prove that I am still worth something to society, to myself. It is important to me that I can still contribute something. Even if it means opening my soul and letting everyone inside. Something I have never done before. The critics say again and again that the book is personal and they are right. Personal. The last shreds of my personal resources. I thought it was important for people to know exactly what it is like to cope with anger, fear and the loneliness of this illness that is murdering my mind. One review said that "The book is an inspiring account of a man of acceptance, wisdom and faith who is 'fighting the good fight' with the hallmark grace and humor of the truly brave."

Should I tell them that I don't feel brave? Most of the time I feel like a scared rat that has just been caught in a trap. I am sure that rat is thinking, I don't want no more of that cheese. I just want out of this son-of-a-bitch." Heartwarming words, nevertheless.

I went back to the Doctors for my monthly check. Little change, so back to the cabin to think and write. I have taken to eating a lot of finger food lately. I can't seem to hit my mouth with a spoon anymore. I look like a two-year old when I am finished eating with a spoon. More food on my lap and on my face than goes into my mouth APRAXIA? Hamburgers and French fries aren't bad though and while I am eating, no one can tell that I can't use a spoon.

I am always exhausted after the drive to the cabin. It was getting late that afternoon when I arrived. The trees were all bare with the exception of the cedar and pines that dot the mountainside. The cabin looked great to me, although every-thing seemed to have changed shape since I was here last. I spent the next hour or so getting re-oriented to every-thing, then unpacked the box of things I had brought with me. There was dust on the floor. I would have to clean that up as soon as I hauled in some firewood. If I would have known that I was going to live this long, I would not have let the maid go.

I thought when I got the diagnosis, that I would die before I made it home from the Doctor's office. Or, in the alternative, be in a nursing home within a week or so. Such was the stereotype Alzheimer's patient that I had seen on TV. It didn't happen quite that way. I know there have been many changes in my life, my personality. How many? I don't know. I am looking for the answers to these questions that bother me still.

As I mentioned before, one of the first signs that can signal the onset of a demanding illness is almost always memory loss. It is only when memory loss, reasoning, orientation etc. can no longer be ignored that medical help is sought. Behavior, as with the gradual withdrawal from friends and social events, will become more obvious. I know that things I once like to do with friends such as fishing and the like, would find me making excuses not to do. Not content to sit and watch TV like before, I would go outside and pace. None of these things by themselves would be any cause for alarm and not be perceived as problematic right away.

All of these things are complicated by the fact that I function very well in soci-ety. It seems I say the right things in a conversation with someone when it is obvi-ous to people that know me well that I have no concept of what is being said. I have told this time and time again.

While on the *ANGELA HILL SHOW* with Dr. Strub, that I mentioned above, I remember hearing Dr. Strub saying, "Most of my Alzheimer's patients don't even know there is a problem. In a way, that can be good." Further he stated, a woman might bring her husband in because of all the problems I have before mentioned. "There is not a damn things wrong with me." He would say and go to his grave without admitting there was a problem. While Larry, on the other hand, knows that he has a problem and he has started writing about the things that are happening to him. He shares them with us and that is a good thing. Every Doctor in the world should read his book. It will give us a better understanding of this disease from the patient's point of view."

You wouldn't know it to look at me now, but at one time I had it all. The Cadillac's, the swimming pool, the 50-foot sloop with fore and aft mainsails. A mainsail and a jib, actually, the shaggy "Joe" dog that lived to catch a ball or lean on my leg when I came home from work. All of that is gone now. Not gone really, but does not have the same meaning as before. We saved for our Golden Years, my wife, Nancy and I. She has been dead for a long time now. My daughter says that she is losing me by the inch. What good is the money now? Other than just enough to live on. To pay for my nursing home or give to some doctor that tells you not come back anymore, there is nothing more he can do for me? To hell with all of that. Take that cruise. Buy that 100 dollar Sergio Valente shirt. Buy it if you want it. Enjoy it. You may be able to remember that you once had it. Build those memories that you can call on.

I really don't mind a doctor telling me he does not know what to do or where to send me for further help. They just don't know. I recognize the inherent limitation of available treatment. They can only treat on the basis of what is scientifically known at this time. However I must say that available treatments are slowly becoming more available. I do resent being talked down to. I am not a dummy. Crazy perhaps, but not stupid. On one of my good days, I can still use words that will send most anyone to the dictionary. On the bad days, I can't from a complete sentence. I say things like, "I want something freezer to drink" or, "I have just been sitting here looking out the mirror, etc."

Fortunately, everyone at the Drug Study program at Ochsners couldn't treat me better. They answer all my questions in words that anyone can understand. They treat me with the utmost respect. Sometimes they die laughing at some of the answers I give them to questions that are on the mental status tests.

"What was the last holiday that we observed?" they asked.

"Jazz fest!" I answered. They died laughing. I don't think they have ever had another patient quite like me.

I can remember listening to a radio talk show one time. There was a doctor talking the calls. One caller called to ask how they should talk to their Alzheimer's patient. She told the caller to talk to her patient like he was a five-year old. That would be painting all Alzheimer's patients with the same brush. That statement is not fair to me and the hundreds of other patients just like me. There may be a day when her statement is true and would be necessary, but not today. I have said it before, "when you have seen one Alzheimer's patient, you have seen ONE Alzheimer's patient. We are all different.

I have done a hundred talk shows about the book, why I wrote it and the like. One question keeps comin up. "How can you be sure you have Alzheimer's?" I have developed a standard answer. "I am not at all sure. It seems to be the doctors that are sure. I just think that my planets are just out of whack or that I probably got bit by a tsetse fly. I didn't diagnose myself. I had some of the best doctors in the United States. They were the ones that made the diagnosis. Ten or twelve of them. I am hoping, of course, that they are all wrong. I still cling to the hope that they all made a mistake and that I have something that is treatable."

I may be running non-empty, but I am still running. I laugh, I cry, I love, I want, I need and I hope. I move about and really enjoy chatting with people. Even the Doctors will tell you that's a life. You see, I am not that much different from you.

It is harder on Stella, I think. She cannot plan anything too far in advance. She says that I don't fit into a niche and stay there. I keep going in and out. Just because I am straight right now doesn't mean that I will be tomorrow.

Have I sat on the pity pot? The answer is yes. Sometimes I feel cheated out of the things I wanted to do when I got older. I will never have a 50th wedding anniversary like my Mom and Dad did. I feel abuse sometimes; at some of the remarks people feel they need to say when they see me on a bad day; i.e. an old drunk, an escapee from the nuthouse. Dispiriting emotions? I have had them all at one time or another.

I have said before that Alzheimer's is an expensive disease. A fellow from a Radio station in Chicago was inter-viewing me. It came up in the conversation that I left my organization because I was making mistakes on inventory. Not returning phone calls, etc. "I can't believe that a mistake or two on inventory should be cause for leaving your job, he said.

"It is quite different than you think," I said. "We handled Oil field Explosives and the State as well as the ATF have strict guidelines on inventory, either or both will come and check your records from time to time. If there is anything not exactly right, according to their guidelines, they will give you a Ticket. Not unlike a traffic ticket."

Then: "I got one at one time for having the wrong number on a roll of prima-cord (Detonating Fuse) inventory. I had a spool number on the inventory sheet rather than the day shift code that they require. It made no difference that I only had one roll and there was no way to get it mixed up with others. If it were to have been stolen, I think I would have known it right away." A thousand-dollar fine.

Another time one of the padlocks on the Explosive locker was one millimeter too small. A coat of paint would have made it legal. Another thousand-dollar fine. "It is my opinion that they have people writing their guidelines that would not know a roll of prima-cord from a spool of rope. But when they started making these violations subject to imprisonment, I got out of the business. You must understand though, I didn't know at that time that I had Alzheimer's. I just thought I must have too much to do and needed to pay more attention to detail. Anyway this disease has cost me a fortune before I knew I had it. In my case, Alzheimer's has shamefully enriched the crown state of Louisiana. I had to quit. Don't you see?"

I must drive my friends half-crazy sometimes with my silly questions. "What time is it? What day is it?" Even, "What year is it?" Or just for fun, "How many solders in the Swiss Army do you suppose carry Swiss Army Pocket Knives?"

I have been spending more time than ever at the Cabin. Stella still calls two or three times a week. Last night when she called, I said, "It sure is cold here, Stel. Bonnie said that it was 10 below zero. I don't care what the scientists say, I support global warming."

Later in the conversation she said that I sounded worried about something. She can always tell. Actually I was worried about a TV show that I was scheduled to do in Fayetteville the next Monday. It was below Zero and the roads were covered with snow, but I told her, "Yes, there is something that has been bothering me for some time."

"What?"

"Where am I going to hang my Pulitzer?" I asked.

"Oh, is that all?" she said with a laugh. "You haven't won yet."

"You sound like you have some doubts, Stell. You need to have faith. That's okay. I have enough for both of us."

"You always were a dreamer, Larry. I hope your wildest dreams come true," she said.

She called again just before I would have to leave for Fayetteville. I was feeling good about the TV thing. The roads were clear now and it was a little warmer. Armed with the AUTOMAP and an Arkansas map, I drove without incident to the interview. I checked off each town and crossroads as I passed them. No problem. Kelly Kemp, the lady that was doing the interview, had given me good directions to the studio. I got there about an hour before the time for the show so I walked around the nearby mall for a while.

I checked in with the receptionist a little while before airtime. She smiled, as she must have recognized me. She said, "We have a book around here somewhere that has a picture of a fellow on the back that looks just like you."

"He must be a really handsome due, Huh?" I asked.

"Sure enough. Would that handsome dude like some coffee while you wait?" she asked.

"Hey, that would be just great. I love my coffee. I have never turned down a cup of coffee in my life. I don't believe that I have been getting enough in my diet lately."

"Great. I will get you some in our new 'Channel 5' cup and you can keep it when you go," she said proudly.

"That's great. You don't mind if I take two, do you?"

"Uh...No, I guess not."

"No way," I said. "I was just joking with you. Perhaps a little Alzheimer's humor there."

Kelly met me in the lobby. We went over what questions she was going to ask me on the show. At last, it was time.

The program went well, I thought. We talked a little about the disease, then people could call in with questions. When the half-hour show was over, there were still some folks wanting to talk to me, so the receptionist took the numbers and I returned all the calls. Later, we were all gathered in the lobby talking. There was several of the production crew there. The weatherman, a couple of cameramen, Kelly, and others.

"You know, of all the places I could have built a mountain cabin, I thank God every day that I built it here in the Arkansas Ozarks," I said. "The people here are so warm and friendly, eager to help you out. I would like to personally thank very man, woman, and child that live here. If I live long enough."

"Larry, I don't think you understand, "said the receptionist. "The people here are your friends because you are one first. You have a smile that could melt Chocolate. People anywhere will treat you pretty much the way you treat them."

I am sure what she said was true but seems to me the hill people here are different. "I must be getting back to the cabin," I told them. Kelly asked if I wanted to get something to eat before I left. I said no, that I was not hungry right then. That I would stop and get a hamburger down the road. I didn't want to embarrass her in case I dribbled food all over myself. She followed me outside to make sure I could find my truck.

"It's right over there," I said, pointing to the truck.

"Where?" she asked.

"The purple one, right over there. No.... Not purple, some other color." I pointed to my truck. "There."

"Yes, I see it," she said. She watched while I drove away to make sure that I was headed in the right direction. I made it back to the cabin without any problems. I built up the fire and sat on the couch. There were a lot of phone calls to return. I would do that later. It wasn't long before I fell asleep.

The phone ringing woke me up. It was Kelly, making sure I had made it home all right. "The show was just great, Larry. Everyone wants you to come back later and do another one. Our phone has been ringing off the hook."

"Sure, I would be happy to do that, but lets wait until it gets a little warmer. Okay?"

"Sure, I'll call you to set it up. We would like to have Stella with you next time, if you can make it," she said.

We chatted awhile longer than hung up. I was feeling good. Remembering what Dr. Strub had told me about thinking more clearly when one is feeling good about himself. I am becoming an advocate for Alzheimer's disease whether I want to or not, it seems.

The more I am able to learn about this disease, the more I realize how little is known or how differently each Doctor explains it to me. If you were like I was before Alzheimer's struck, I knew very little. What I have found out since is that most if the information is often incorrect. The disease is not a mental illness or psychological disorder, but rather a physical disorder cause by the destruction of nerve cells in specific areas of the brain.

There may be a number of causes. Some of the suggested causes are so speculative that they belong in the realm of science fiction, i.e. Aluminum, slow viruses such as the rare Kuru and as we mentioned earlier, Creutzfeldt-Jacobs. How odd. I just learned the Creutzfeldt-Jacobs is certainly related to what is called the "Mad Cow" disease. That you can possibly get from eating beef, so far limited to England. They may have to kill over 12 million cows in order to wipe out that cause.

Dr. Allen Roses has stated that he has found a gene or a genetic defect that could account for early onset Alzheimer's. He has also decided that it might be possible the cause is entirely different than anything suggested so far. Only continued research and study will answer these questions.

I drove to Branson the next day, using the same technique as I did going to Channel 5. Just to see if I could do it again. I don't worry about getting lost much anymore. No one stays lost forever. I have found that I must stay alert. If I let my mind wander for a moment, I have a tough time getting back to where I was before. I still have a pretty good sense of direction. At night, I can still find the dipper in the stars. Then the North Star. No problem, if I just think; I can do it.

Not long ago, Stella and I were in Missouri, coming back to the cabin from a book signing. I was driving. I knew I was on the right road. I don't remember the Highway Number right now, but I knew at the time that it was the right one.

Suddenly I got the feeling that I was going North rather than South to Arkansas. I told Stella, "I think we are going the wrong direction."

"I can't help you," she said. "I don't have any idea where we are." She had been dozing. By the time I slowed down to turned around, I got straightened out again. It was like the whole world had just whirled around and I was going right again. I don't know how that sort of things happens. I don't recall it ever happening again.

On that same trip, we were also in western Kansas near where I once lived. I decided to go past my wife's grave and say 'Hello' to her. I don't like to go there in the winter because it is so cold and desolate there. I hate to think of her being there in the ice and snow. I stopped at a store in town and bought her a stuffed dog. She loved dogs. Any kind. She loved them all. It must have taken us an hour to find her grave. I knew I was on the right lane, but I thought it was further back into the cemetery than I remembered. I finally found it and placed the dog behind the headstone and said something, I don't' remember what. Stella was with me. She asked if I wanted to be alone for a moment.

"No, I guess not Stel. You know, I can't even remember what she looked like. She was blonde. I remember that." We walked back to the car in silence.

14

Memory Problems

While I was out driving somewhere, I think I was coming back from the trip to Branson that I mentioned a few pages back, my thought returned to just getting to the cabin. I checked the map. I was in familiar territory now. I drove on down the road looking out the windshield at nothing in particular. My thoughts had drifted away for a while, but had no ill effect on my destination. I stopped at a little food store not far from the cabin and picked up a few things to eat, then drove on home.

It was really cold, so I turned on the heat pump while I built a fire in the wood stove. It wasn't long before it was getting not. I turned off the heat pump and stood near the potbelly. A motion out the back window facing the hollow caught my attention. A deer, perhaps, I turned for a better look. My elbow touched the stovepipe. Burned like hell. It seems I am always burning myself lately. Last night I turned on the range to heat up a can of soup and I just realized, it is still on. All night and all day? Got to be more careful. Seems like I tell myself that every hour.

While I am painfully aware that my condition is a real problem, I keep reassuring myself that the disease is quiescent right now. That I have reached that plateau. If plateau is the right word, Still I find it hard and harder to do the things that I could do just last year. My first book was written without too much difficult. This one is making me work. I seem to get bogged down over a word or phrase that takes me all day to get right.

Sometimes I may write a thought or an idea, then wonder where it came from. Was that my thought or did I just hear it on the TV or read it somewhere. I would never want to write down someone else's thought or idea without giving them the credit. Should I preface every thing with "I heard somewhere" or "I read somewhere?" It takes me a lot of more time.

The publisher called a while ago asking how the writing was going.

"You know, Susan, I had some great thoughts while driving this morning. Thoughts to put in the book. They were so simple and straightforward that I didn't use the tape recorder that I keep in the seat beside me. Now that I am ready to write, I haven't a clue what the thoughts were all about. Not a clue, I just can't seem to get them back."

"Use the recorder, Larry, or stop the car and write it down on a note pad like you did before. Make a habit of doing that. You will do okay," she said.

Do I really want to admit that I have an illness that is affecting my memory? I know it to be true, but I keep telling myself that it will soon stop. One of the Doctors said that I was still in denial. The cold hard facts are that I am losing my memory and it won't come back. Sometimes it does, but most of the time it does not. What is the harm in delaying reality?"

Friends say, "I am going to tell you the truth." But they don't tell you the truth. They say things like, "I wouldn't worry. You seem all right to me." or "You're not as young as you used to be." or "You are just slowing down a little."

I hope they are right, but I know they are not. The realization that you will not ever recover can be very frightening. You think, "What will I do? What can I do?" Well, you do all you can for as long as you can, is what I would say.

When Stella asked one of the Doctors that first diagnosed me what should she let me do. He said, "Don't fence Larry in. Let him do anything that he thinks he can do. Don't make an invalid out of him." So far Stella has never forgotten what the doctor told her. In fact, she encourages me to do all that I can. Although I mowed the grass three times last week. It is winter and the grass isn't growing, she cheers me on, telling me what a good job I have done.

At one period of time, she worried about me driving alone to the cabin, but lately she has taken the attitude that I have, that no one stays lost forever. Someone will find me. She may worry, but she doesn't let on. I have a phone in my truck now that if ever needed, I just say, "Call Stella" and it does it. Isn't technology great? I have never had to use it (yet) in such an emergency. Hope I never do.

I mentioned a few pages back about visiting my late wife's grave. There is a place for me there beside her. I have a place to go to. I have been thinking about that unpleasant eventuality lately. I have just about decided to donate all of my organs to the medical community; if there is anything left that will be of use to anyone. The eyes will still be good, I am sure. It does my heart good to think of someone being able to use these old eyes. A teen-aged girl, for instance, to be able to see her date at the high school prom or for a little boy, perhaps, to be able to see how to bait a hook. What a gift. What a gift that would be and all because of me. Think of it that way. You can't be sad.

I don't know how old a person has to be before they won't take your heart anymore. If anyone can use it, they are welcome. It is a good heart. Ask anyone that knows me. The liver, kidneys, anything else that can be used. Take all that is good and the junk that is left, just burn it and throw it to the wind. I will have already achieved a certain degree of immortality.

I have made a videotape of what I want when the times comes for me to go. I have spelled it out exactly what I want and I don't want anyone taking part of it out of context. I don't want to do myself in because of the reasons I have just mentioned above. It might be a time before anyone finds me and by that time none of the organs would be any value to anyone. I have said that I want no one to go to any heroic efforts or do anything to prolong my life if I happen to be in a hospital or nursing home, etc. If anyone, a Doctor, Judge, DA, Right to Life do-gooders, Congress, or any other son-of-a-bitch group, does anything to prolong my life when it is no longer a quality life, I want whoever is my guardian at that time to sue the bastards for every penny they have. That is what I want when the time comes. I hope it is another twenty years.

15

A Sad Story

Today I got a letter from a girl I California. It was one of the saddest letters I have ever received. She had just read my book. She said she was reading everything she could get her hands on about Alzheimer's. It seems that her boyfriend had developed all of the symptoms overt the last couple of years. Some of the same things that happened to me were happening to him. Even more. She said that he had been forgotten which handle was hot and which was cold in the shower. He went through all the same tests that I did. The diagnosis…Alzheimer's. The man is 36.

I can't write everyone back that writes to me about the book. It would keep me busy day and night. Don't think that I don't appreciate the letters though. I read and reread every one of them and I keep them as well. But, I wrote this lady back at once. I gave her my home telephone number just in case she ever needed to talk to someone. As desperate as my situation is, hers it seems, is even more desperate.

I haven't had any trouble with the water faucets yet. I can still remember the old saying about what it takes to be a Master Plumber. "Hot on the left, cold on the right, crap run downhill and payday is on Friday."

Speaking of left and right, my son always tell me, especially when I am getting ready to go on the road somewhere, Dad, if you don't remember anything else, for God's sake remember, the left lane is the fast lane, and the right lane is the slow lane."

One more of his words of wisdom is as follows: "Dad, you only need two things get by, as far as tools are concerned. You need WD-40 and Duct tape. If it doesn't move and it should; use the WD-40. If it moves and it shouldn't; use the Duct tape.

16

Rating Scales & Chat Rooms

This must be an exciting time for those scientists and medical personnel who are researching Alzheimer's disease. Only a few short years ago, there were only a few who were interested in this problem. We will all agree that Alzheimer's was far removed from the interests and skills of the medical profession. Now, it seems that everyone is jumping on the bandwagon. It couldn't be soon enough to suit me. None of us can conquer this disease alone. By working closely with the medial profession, we are doing something about it. Not only the patient is of interest to the medical people, but there is also new interest in coping for the caregivers. They are a lonely lot only a few years ago. Now there are support groups in virtually every major city in the United States.

Nursing homes around the U.S. are working on how to give better care for their Alzheimer's patients. Special care units to better serve the needs of the mentally impaired patients are springing up all over. I see it almost weekly on TV.

There is still so much about Alzheimer's that is not understood. And maybe never will be. There is still no single best way to treat every patient, but more; and more is being learned every day. Are these 'Medical Breakthroughs' real or imaginary? Only time will tell. Treatment is still somewhat limited.

You see ads on TV most every day about a man being embarrassed by Toenail Fungus. In all of my life, I have never heard of Toenail Fungus. The ads make it look like everyone in the U.S. has it and doesn't know what to do about it. It makes me want to throw a brick through the TV screen. If the only problem I had was Toenail Fungus, I think I could live a perfectly normal life.

When your spouse, or someone you love, has been diagnosed with Alzheimer's. Like most folks, you know very little about this disease. You have seen patients on TV in the worst possible condition. You have heard just enough to be afraid. Join the crowd. The nursing home picture is what you expect. You have questions, but you are afraid to ask. You are not sure you even want to know. The person you have relied upon for five years is forgetful, confused and becoming increasingly dependent on you. He or She is given to unpredictable mood changes, once quite foreign to you. You have a million questions and don't quite know what to do next. Again, let me say, contact the Alzheimer's Association as soon as possible. They can start you on the right path. There are many Government agencies in your own community that can also help you. Also, read, read, and read. There are many books on the subject now days that were not available when I was first diagnosed. You don't need to believe everything you read. Much of what I have read is 100% wrong. Make up your own mind. Use what will work for you. WE can all only hope that prevention and treatment is near.

Denial will be the first form of not accepting the diagnosis. You will think that everyone is wrong and that you are just depressed or distracted. This stage is temporary. You will begin to develop an inner awareness. You may become angry at the unfairness of this disease. That too will pass. Anger is normal, in my view, because you are losing control of your life and there is nothing you can do about it. Where do you aim your anger? Who or what will be your target? God? Your caregiver? The Doctors? Such anger will only make you feel guilty. Get over this stage. Concentrate on something else. Go pet your pig. Anything, until this mood passes. As time goes by, the anger may continue, but you will begin to feel more control, more accepting of this change in your lifestyle.

A few days ago, I had a call from a young lady in graduate school that wanted my help on her dissertation on Alzheimer's She said that she had read the book and asked if I could give her any more information about the disease. She said that my input would carry a great deal of weight in the academic community because of my writings.

I told her that I would be happy to help her. I would do anything and everyone possible to further the research of Alzheimer's. "I don't take myself too seriously about the weight that my writings may have, however." I told her. "I may get a year of two of celebrity, a starring role in some academic papers, a talk show or two and then shoved away in some nursing facility where I will be cared to death. Just another statistic."

Further, there are Functional Rating Scales that can be obtained from your Doctors or from the Alzheimer's Association. Your caregiver can circle the highest number response which best describes your behavior. Then compare with the last ones. Below are a few of the questions that may be found on your Rating scale. There are several different ones but they all work about the same way. The caregiver can pick the ones they like. This one is from Hutton, Dippel, Loewenson, Mortimer and Christians, 1985. They may have an updated version by now.

The latest Functional Rating Stella filled out for me is as follows:

Eating:	Eats messily, has some difficulty with utensils.
Dressing:	Able to dress self with occasional mismatched socks. Needs supervision with buttons and laces.
Continence:	Complete control
Verbal Commendation:	Difficulties with word finding. Able to carry out simple uncomplicated conversation.
Names:	Remembers names of meaningful acquaintances.
Events:	Cannot recall details or sequences of recent events.
Mental Alertness:	Alert
Confusion:	Periodic confusion during daytime.
Orientation:	Oriented, usually able to find his bearings.
Recognition:	Can recognize faces of recent acquaintances.
Hygiene and Grooming:	Usually neat and clean.
Emotionality:	Moderate change in emotional responsiveness. growing apathy, increased rigidity, despondent, unstable, laughs or cries in inappropriate situations.
Social responsiveness:	has a tendency to dwell in the past, lack of proper association for present situation. Antisocial at times.
Sleep Patterns:	Sleeps more or less normal.

Be creative in finding sources of support. Effort is being made by political advocates of Alzheimer's victims in finding ways to aid patients for as long as possible in their homes. There are care centers now in a lot of the major cities that provide the caregivers needed respites. If your patient is a Veteran, the VA may be of help. The caregivers need not be overwhelmed. Make use of these facilities. It is a means to an end.

Any caregiver can tell you that support groups have been found to be quite helpful in problem solving and education about the disease as well as providing emotional support. You can learn from everyone there, I am told. There is also getting to be a large number of Chat Rooms on the Internet for caregivers. There you can talk to folks from all over the world. I was instrumental in creating a Web Site. It is DASN.com (Dementia advocates support network) Now there is DASNI.com (international) Just type in DASN or DASNI into your search engine. Go there and you will find links to chat rooms. One good one we use right now is alzinfo.org You can learn much by clicking on their site.

As I said, there is a group of Alzheimer's patients that I chat with from time to time. There must be 15 or 20 patients from all over the world. Most are about my age, some younger. We all try to help each other with the problems that we may be having on a particular day. Compare treatments. We support each other when one of us is down. Things like that. One can draw strength from everyone there.

This is a lonely disease. You gradually lose your friends and eventually your family as well. Anger and fear is also part of Alzheimer's. There is an old saying: Keep your words sweet in case you have to eat them. I find myself distancing myself from the social life. I am just as content to sit and listen to music or watch TV, or just staring at nothing in particular. I have found that if you are stressed, you imagine yourself in a peaceful place. Sitting on Bayou bank fishing, or out in the woods, or on a mountaintop where you can see forever.

The poet, Dillon Thomas, wrote; Do not go gentle into that goodnight; Rage, rage against the dying of the light."

One can rage, but the light is dying. A little each day. There is nothing I can do to stop it. I can dream and imagine. Dream of a time not long ago when there were not enough hours in the day to do all that I wanted. I often wished there was a couple more hours in a day. Crazy, Huh? But life was exciting. Everyday was a new adventure. I was alive, vital, gifted. Those days are gone forever.

Wasn't it Albert Einstein that wrote, "Imagination is more important than knowledge. Knowledge is limited where imagination embraces the entire world. You don't need a map to get there. You can go anywhere, do anything, as long as you are going and doing it in your head."

Not long ago, I saw a program on CNN about Alzheimer's. Again, Dr. Allen Roses, at Duke University, talked a little about his research with Alzheimer's. He said that never in the history of any disease has so much been learned in such a short time. Further he thinks that within a decade, and more than a year, there will be a prototype treatment for this disease. He thinks that within twenty years, Alzheimer's will be a rare disease that may affect only a few people over eighty. His words give us hope where before there was none.

One would be well advised to remember that a great deal of media attention has been generated on Alzheimer's research in the past year or so that have raised hopes only to have them dashed. The most recent is the drug TACRIN. The drug created quite a stir a year or so ago with reports suggesting miraculous bene-fits. Later studies determined that it produced only small temporary improvement and only in a limited number of patients. At least it was something. One small step ahead.

There is one great problem with evaluating therapy, I am told, is the nature of the disease. Unlike other diseases, Alzheimer's lacks any markers other than neuropsychological tests to detect changes in cognitive function. It is my understanding that my being involved in the drug studies for so long a time does this. They compare test scores that are taken every month to the test scores taken before the study began and by comparing those test scores with the drug and placebo treated patients.

In my view there is a problem. A person's cognitive abilities can fluctuate daily or even hourly. It is the natural course of Alzheimer's. Is a change for the better due to the drug or simply that the patient is having a good day? One can only hope that it is the treatment.

I read the HOPE is a way to cope. It is almost impossible to have hope and be a pessimist at the same time. Hope keeps you forging ahead. Hope is power. It is the kind of power that will lead us down a different path, if the one we are on is leading us nowhere. We all know that no matter what our mind is telling us, hope is in your hearts. Listen to your heart, and chant the beauty of the good things in life. Choose to hope, live peacefully, think positively, be optimistic and thank God. Good advice. I should take it myself.

I heard a great story one time on imagination and optimism. It is a story about two men who shared a room at a nursing home. One man, near the door, was blind and completely paralyzed. He couldn't even move his head. His roommate, an old man, had the bed near the window.

Day after day, the blind man would ask his roommate to look out the window and tell him what was happening in the world outside. Time after time the old man by the window would tell his friend what was going on outside in great detail.

He would describe the activity of the people going by. With great spirit, he would report the activities of the mailman, perhaps wearing a coat on a cold day and a short sleeve shirt on the better days. Other things like the volume of mail on certain days and so on. He would talk in great detail about young lovers walking down the sidewalk holding hands. He would describe the traffic, the color of the cars and trucks. The Cadillac has gone too far with style this year, he would say. He would describe a mother bird nesting in the tree right outside the window and report each day on the progress of the young birds until they at last flew away on their own.

The paralyzed man truly lived for the stories of what was going on in the world outside. One day, however, his friend dies. His eyes to the world were lost to him. Later he was assigned a new roommate. Before long the blind man asked his new friend to look out the window and tell him what was going on outside.

"Sure," said the new man. Then:" I don't know how I can. You see, there is nothing outside this window but a brick wall."

How differently two people's perspective on life can be. Some can see the beauty in anything, while others remain oblivious to beauty or kindness.

That story reminds me of a man I met one time named "Hans." Hans was a soldier in the German army in World War Two. I spent hours listening to Hans talk about his experiences in the war. He was quick to tell me that his name was not pronounced "Hawns" but more like you would say "Hands."

Hans drove a tank on the eastern front when they were invading Russia. It seems that an incentive from the command had been given that anyone capturing a Russian tank, intact, would be given a reward of near a thousand dollars. Hans said that he and his crew awoke one morning surrounded by forty or fifty Russian tanks. He just knew that this would be the end for him that he was going to die. His gunner looked at him, smiled and said, "Just look out there at all those tanks, Hans. We're rich."

I believe that was just a story, but it was a great story. It shows how differently two people in the same situation sees things. Could it be that any two Alzheimer's patients (or caregivers) may see things as differently as Hans and his gunner? No matter how we see things, we must fight every moment to have hope and be optimistic.

I was talking with Betty Lou, a retired teacher I had met at the swimming pool at the Country club. "You are quite famous, Larry. Almost everyone I know has read your book. Even some friends that I know in North Carolina have a copy." Eventually the conversation drifted to how we act now and how we acted as a child.

Can you remember when we were small children? Our life was full of wonder, adventure and excitement. We slept only when we could not stay awake any longer. 'We ate only when our mother's made us and we had more energy than our parents could stand. Somewhere along the line, we lost that boundless energy and enthusiasm for life. We tell ourselves that we don't have the energy to do the things we once did. We have somehow lost much of our strength and vitality.

Ask yourself, if when you were a child, you had that boundless energy, why not now? The answer must be in the way a child goes at life. A child lives for the moment. Whereas, we are thinking about the future or the past, and unless we are doing something pleasant, we don't think much about now. We are caught up in working and making a living. Perhaps we could learn a great deal that we have forgotten from watching a child. Although their interests are limited, you can watch them doing their thing with complete joy and wonder. They see everything, hear everything with a curious mind and a joy filled heart. If you don't think they hear everything, just try using one of those four letter words that you don't want them saying. See how quickly the child picks it up. If only we could train ourselves to live as a child does, for this moment, we could be as happy as they.

We say, "Well, we just don't have any interest in things anymore. Life is boring. Too ordinary. We have too many things on our mind." When one says he or she is bored, it doesn't say much for one's character.

Unless we know everything there is to know about everything, there must be something that is of interest to us. Sit down; make a list of things you want to learn all there is to know about. It doesn't make any difference what is on that list. The fact that you were able to write something down shows that you still have an interest. Learn about those things on your list. Learn everything you can about them. Know the benefits and the pitfalls. You will be a better person for it.

As out talk continued, I told Betty Lou, "I have a met and talked with kids, right here at this pool, High School graduates, that have never heard of The Ottoman Empire, Charlemagne, Garibaldi, or even the Magna Carte. I don't remember if I learned about these things in school or not, but I know about them. Can you live your whole life that way or does it make any difference in the end?"

She said, "You can live your life that way, but look at what you would be missing." I have always told the children I taught to "Learn, learn about everything you can, it is the only answer."

There may be additional benefits to learning. Researchers have found that a larger number of people with Alzheimer's are poorly educated. It would appear that education actually might encourage neurons to grow. If this were true, an educated person could lose more neurons without much noticeable change in mental function. In fact, it could possibly delay the onset of the disease. I wish someone would do an in-depth study of this phenomenon. It could prove very interesting.

If we keep our minds, our eyes, our ears and our hearts open, what we may find is the energy and zest for life that our neighbor has. You know the ones that are never bored or listless, the ones that are always doing something with that ageless enthusiasm for life. We all envy them, but we can do it too, once we go at life like that child we were talking about earlier. You have all seen them or raised them. You can be like them. Glad to be alive, eager to discover the wonderful things that are all about us. This may be the one reason that I am still doing fairly well. I never did really grow up. I still haven't decided what I want to be. A rancher, a farmer? Maybe even a bartender…I've got it. A Maytag repairman.

Things puzzle me that didn't bother me before. Like; "What is a round steak?" How about the phrase; "Legally drunk?" If it's legal, what's the problem? What do you say when someone, usually a grandmother at my age, shows you a picture of a really ugly baby. You can't say it is really cute and be truthful. I am afraid I will say something like, "What do they feed it?"

17

Sailing

My son, Jeff, called me from Belize. He and a lady friend had taken the boat down there for some R and R. When they were ready to come back, he discovered that the navigation equipment was on the blink. He didn't want to take a chance on sailing back across the Gulf of Mexico with only a compass. He asked if I would come down there and sail back with them.

I told him, sure, it would be good to get away for a while and spend some time with him. I told him to take the boat up to Cozumel. An easy sail from Belize, and wait for me there. I would meet him at the airport. It is easy to get a flight to Cozumel. Not so easy to go straight to Belize. Stella made the reservations from New Orleans and let Jeff know about what time I should get to he airport there.

I got on the Plane without any trouble. As we were waiting our turn to take off, the pilot came on the speaker and aid, "Welcome to the Golden Gate Flight. We will be stopping briefly in San Francisco and then on to Hawaii." I just about panicked. How in Hell did I manage to get on the wrong plane? I unbuckled my seat belt and was starting up the isle with all the Flight Attendants in pursuit when they finally convinced me that the pilot was only joking, and that we were indeed going to Cozumel. We would be there in one hour and twenty minutes. If the Airline crew only knew how close I came to throwing a fit. Did you ever see anyone have a conniption? That is what my Mother called it. It is not pretty. Oh, you don't have a conniption, you pitch one.

True to his word, the plane soon landed in Cozumel. The Emerald waters of the Caribbean always take your breath away. This time was no exception. Jeff and his friend met me just past customs.

"Dad, meet my; very good friend, Dr. Elizabeth Smith. She is from Denver."

"My, I said, how pretty you are Elizabeth. Did I hear Jeff say you were also a Doctor? I am certainly looking forward to coming down with an affliction that would require your services."

"Sorry, Mr. Rose, I am a gynecologist."

"Just my luck, and please I am just Larry. When someone says Mr. Rose, I start looking for my dad."

"Okay, your call."

"Anything you want to do while you are here Dad?"

"I guess not. I have had all the fun I can stand for one day. Where did you put the boat?"

"It's at Puerto de Abrigo. Just a short walk from here, or we could take taxi. It's only a buck." Jeff said. "We have a lot of food on the boat. Enough for a week or more. Do you want to cook something there or eat here before we go? The Hotel Mara and Hotel Cantarell is just across the beach from the boat, if you want to get something to eat there."

"I don't care. I'll just follow you guys," I said.

"What is the matter with the Navigation equipment?"

"I don't know Dad. That is the reason I called the pro."

"Well, did you kick it?"

"No, Dad. I don't do things like that anymore."

"They tell me you should try kicking it. Get the rotors and servos going." I said.

"Do you remember that sign you had on the radar at one time; the one that looked like it was written in German?"

"Yes, I remember the ACHTUNG one?"

"That is the one. I took is seriously." he said with a smile.

It went like this:

ACHTUNG ALLES LOOKENSPEEPERS

Das Machine ist not fer gefingerpoken and mittengrabben. Ist easy schnappen der springenwerk, blowenfussen, und poppencorken mit spittzensparken. Ist nicht fer gewrken by das dummkopfen. Das rubberrnecken sightsseeran, keepen der hands in das pockets, relaxen and jas vatch das blinkenlights.

"Right Jeff. I loved that sign. A fellow at Gearhardt Industries in Fort Worth gave that sign to me years ago."

"Let's get underway then, Okay? Glad you are here with us, Dad. It's not easy for just two people to sail this thing. We have a full tank of Diesel, Charts, and a full tank of potable water. We checked the clock with Greenwich Mean Time. We have everything we should need."

We checked our location a couple of time, finding we were 6 hours west of Greenwich, 90 degrees and a couple of minutes. Right on course. Jeff joked that we should reach the U.S. somewhere between Mobile Bay and Houston.

"Close enough." I told him.

We had no problems. Jeff didn't really need me along. He would ask me a question now and then. Questions that I sure he already knew. He was just trying to make me feel useful, I think. I pray I will never forget that trip. We had fun. We were not father and son on that trip. We were pals.

18

Some Things to Watch out for

I am asked continually, on radio and TV talk shows, what advice could you give someone that may have just been diagnosed with Alzheimer's? That is the toughest question. What works for me may not work for someone else. I think the best advice for anyone would be to keep busy. Do all of the things that you are capable of doing. Do crossword puzzles, play solitaire. It is a card game that may help keep you counting. Both up and down. Anything like that.

Remember that when you get older, debility is not inevitable. Some public figures remain vigorous well into old age. Some include: May West, Pablo Picasso, Eubie Blake and we all know of Konrad Adenaure as well.

There is some good news. I am told that only about half of all Alzheimer's cases eventually result in the patient becoming incapacitated. So incapacity may not be a problem for all of us. The one main reason this disease is so scary, in my view, is that it will affect the higher functions: Thinking, reasoning, remembering. It is those activities that make us who we are.

Some caveats for the caregivers to remember, remain with one topic at a time. Don't assume your patient can follow rapid conversational transitions. They may become stuck on a word or phrase. Find a way to say it differently, rather than repeating over and over. Avoid long-winded sentences and third person pronouns. Be alert. Your patient may substitute a loosely related word for the one you expect him to use. A cup rather than a glass, or words that sound the same. Pup for cup. Also your patient may know that a dog is a dog and may say it, when asked for the higher order name such as Poodle, etc. may not be able to think of it.

Other things to watch for include:

BURNS: Light bulbs, stoves and so on. I have burns almost all the time. I have no idea where or how I got them.

BED: Getting in and out, tangled blankets or the bed may be too high.

RUGS: Can be slippery, bathtubs as well. You can get non-slip bath mats, non-slip tape for the tub. You may also want to set your water heater down a few degrees to avoid scalds.

STAIRS: Another scary thing for the Alzheimer's patient. I avoid stairs at all cost.

Loud TV. A war show with guns and bombs may be mistaken for the real thing.

KEEP HALLWAYS and your main traveled areas well lit and clutter free to avoid falls We are not as nimble as we once were.

Although it has been some time now since the TWA Flight 800 crash, it continues to make the news now and then in the country's newspapers and stories on TV. Interest in the victims and their families is still on our minds. You can read names of victims in the paper. It doesn't seem to tug at your heart until you see a name you recognize. Dr. Yvon Lamour was such a name for me. He is one of France's leading authorities on Alzheimer's disease, having spent two stints at the National Institute of Health in Washington.

A brilliant researcher and a scientist, the doctor has written a book on Alzheimer's disease and the again of the brain. His book is titled the AGE OF UNREASON. Required reading for everyone in the field. Sad to lose a mind like his.

To all of those who lost a friend or family members in this tragic crash, please know that I too share in your loss. Dr. Lamour may have been the one to find a cure for this disease. Now he is gone as well as the hopes and dreams of all the other passengers.

19

Manners

I knew it would happen one day. As I have said earlier, I have received hundreds of letters from folks all over and felt compelled to let me know what they thought of the book and how it affected them. So far all of the letters were great. Not one derogatory review from anyone. That all changed today. The letter started out good enough, but further on in the letter, she stated that she was confused. That I had stated in the book that I had a relationship with God and that I believed in the Bible's view of him. She stated further that she did not believe what I wrote about my relationship with God because of what she read on page 47. I had to go look at what I had written.

It seems that my good friend Tyrone, had come to my rescue when someone in the café called me an "old drunk" when I had trouble walking through the café. He said he would kick their "God damn ass" all the way to the street. I am sure not going to take anyone to task for what they say or believe especially when they coming to my rescue. If you were in the middle of the ocean, drowning, and a boat came along and someone in the boat threw you a rope, I don't think you would ask about his religion before you grabbed hold.

I am not trying to convince or change anyone. I am just trying real hard to adjust to this Alzheimer's thing.

She went on to say the Bible speaks of knowing God only through his boy, Jesus. I know all of that. At one time I had a real knowledge of the Bible. I'll bet I could stand toe to toe with her when it comes to scripture. One is limited on what you can write in one book about your beliefs on any subject, including the Bible. Maybe I should have explained further.

Her beliefs are great if they work for her. She must be doing everything about right. To me, it is just a matter of manners. I wonder if she realizes that Christianity is a minority in the world. Does this mean that everyone else is destined to go to Hell? I don't think so. I wrote her back, telling her that some Idiot had been writing crazy letters to people and signing her name to them. I thought she should know. (Copy of letter enclosed.)

It seems that manners are getting to be a lost art in American. Manners are always important; from the coffee shops to a job interview. I couldn't tell you, over the years, how many job applicants I have dismissed for the lack of manners. Manners are even more important between friends and lovers. Spouses are particularly important. Manners will show them that they are very important to us and we are away of their feelings and that we enjoy having them around.

I try not to make anyone feel that they are taken for granted. Open that door for a lady. Hold that chair for them and don't stop after today. Make it a part of the real you. And please, do not question anyone's relationship and God when you don't have any idea how he or she really feels.

We have all lost loved ones at sometime in our lives that may have never really know how much we cared for them. Have you told them what a good choice you made by having them involved in your life? Have you tried today to show your spouse that he or she is the only one? If not, do it now. Tomorrow might be too late. In my case, my wife, Nancy, left for work one morning and I never saw her again. As I remember, what I said that morning was "see you later, Babe". Don't let this happen to you, if you really love someone. Tell them now.

We tend to blame our faults and shortcomings on everything from our parents to the stars. My Dad whipped me a couple of times when I was a little guy, but I probably had it coming and I don't hate him for it. I didn't turn out to be a mass murderer. Caesar may have said it best with his quote. "The fault is not in the stars, Dear Brutus, but in ourselves."

20

Stage three?????

I continually ask the doctors, "How much longer do you think I have before I lost it?" Take it from me; they will never discuss your future in great detail. Their reluctance is understandable. It would be virtually impossible to predict how the disease in each person would progress, since the symptoms and rate of progression vary so widely in each case. Some symptoms can show up early in some and not until much later or not at all in other patients. Some develop psychiatric problems. Others never do. For some the decline is gradual, as in my case, while others experience a sharp downhill course ending in death in a very short time.

Dr. Kevin McKinney is one of the great Doctors that work on the drug study at Ochsners. He is young, personable, smart, and a Board Certified Physician in Neurology. He is helping with the study under the aegis of Dr. Strub. He told me that symptoms are influenced by the patient's intellect, personality, coping skills one develops, physical health and of course support from your friends and family. He states further that while there is usually predictable progression from one stage to the next. That is not always the case. A patient may exhibit at one of the early stages, characteristics usually associated with the advance stages or in some cases skip a stage altogether. The progression from stage to stage is seldom neat and smooth.

I receive articles almost daily that someone thinks might be of interest to me. I just got one in the mail from a lady named Linda. Her article is as follows:

"Solvents Associated with increased Alzheimer's" It goes on; "Exposure to solvents such as toluene, trichlo-roethane, and hexane can cause structural changes in neurons and biochemical changes in nerve synapses and neuro-transmitters. They especially affect areas of the brain important in memory and in Alzheimer's disease, such as the hippocampus. When the solvent insult is coupled with other neuronal loss and degeneration due to aging and other factors, the susceptibility to Alzheimer's disease and the likelihood of Alzheimer's disease expression may increase. That is what noted researchers of a case-controlled study investigating solvent exposure and risk of Alzheimer's in a study base of 23,000 persons, aged 60 years or more, taken from membership in a health maintenance organization in Seattle. Washington, have decided that the cumulative brain damage from solvent exposure at a cellular level, or decreased "neuronal reserve" may then allow the accumulation of the brain changes associated with Alzheimer's to reach critical levels more quickly."

The researchers found a relatively strong association between history of solvent exposure to one or more solvent groups (benzene and toluene; phenols and alcohol; ketones; or other solvents), and Alzheimer's disease, with an especially marked elevation in risk for males. Therefore they conclude that past exposure to organic solvents may be associated with the onset of Alzheimer's disease."

Reference:
Kukall, W. A.; Larson, E. B, et al. "Solvent Exposure as a Risk Factor for Alzheimer's Disease: A Case-Control Study." AMERICAN JOURNAL OF EPIDEMIOLOGY 131 (11): 1059-1071 (1995) EARN Library Code: 1494-KUKU-95013R=$3.50…. For more information.

That about covers everything in Stage Three. Stage Four is the tough one. This is the stage where the most dramatic changes occur as the patient progresses toward Stage Five. Language skills gone, memory loss so bad by now that everything is unfamiliar and threatening. My prayer is that I never reach Stage four.

Sometimes I feel like the other shoe is about to fall. Yesterday, I did my wash and forgot to put soap in the machine. I may have never noticed, but as I was loading the dryer, I saw a dirty spot on a golf shirt that didn't come clean. It dawned on me then that I did not use any soap. I must have filled the machine with water, and then got distracted by something else. Another coping thing.

Let's go back a bit to last summer. I just found my notes from June. I was alone at the Cabin. I am spending most of my time there now. My sister, Lois, called to tell me that our old school was having an alumni reunion in a few days and could I come?

"I don't think so Lois. I don't drive so far anymore."

"I will come and get you then if you want to go. And bring you back when you want to go home," she said. "I will even pay for the gas."

"That sounds like a deal, but I am not destitute yet. I still haven't loaded up my Visa. I can surely pay for the gas if you are driving all this way. Hell, I will even buy you a hamburger or a bowl of Chili or something."

"Here I come." she said.

Once back in Kansas, we just hung out for the next day or so. Visiting with friends and neighbors. Then it was time to go to the Alumni thing. Everything gets together in the afternoon and talks over old times, and then at night they have a dinner and dance.

I fit right in. Those days are still vivid in my mind. I ran across an old class-mate, Gary Roland, in the hall. "Hey, Rosie, good to see you, glad your could make it. I have just been talking to our first grade teacher, Miss Jaques. She is in the room down at the end of the hall." I almost ran to the room. I sure wanted to see her. How long has it been? Near fifty years.

She recognized me right away. We chatted for a long time. Memories came flooding back to those days in the first grade. Like putting pennies on the train track. The time Miss Jaques swatted Larry McCue and me on the butt for leaving the school grounds while chasing a boomerang that didn't come back.

"Do you remember when your dog had puppies, and you tried for nine days to give me one of the pups?' she asked me.

"You know, I really don't remember that.' I said.

"I asked you how many pups did she have and you told me, 'bout a million". She said laughing.

"I do remember one time you were standing in the back of the class and you told me to go to your desk and bring you a fork that was there. "AND DON'T BREAK IT". You said. It was a trick fork that had a hinge in the middle. As soon as I picked it up, the tines fell down. I just knew that I had broken it right after you told me not to."

She laughed like crazy. "You haven't changed a bit."

"Yes, I have. Now days I wouldn't try to give you a puppy. I would try to SELL you one."

We looked at old photos of the class. Gary and I even remembered the names of some of the kids that Miss Jaques had forgotten. It was a great afternoon.

I don't remember if I asked her about her husband, Harold Hunt. Harold was my hero when I was 8 or 9 years old. It was right after the war. He owned a business there in our small town. He always had a job for me to do after school Sweep the floor, wash the windows or carry out the trash. Scoop the snow off the side-walk in the wintertime. He would pay me with a bottle of pop and a candy bar. I was the envy of some of the other kids.

Each class gathered in different classrooms. I think ours would have been the class of '55'. About everyone was there. Christine, Judy, Gary, his wife Zo Ann. I think Zo was a year younger. Then there was another childhood friend, Garry Chaffin. I hadn't seen him for at least thirty years. He looked the same. It seemed everyone had old pictures to see and were taking new ones at the same time. We were all talking, laughing and reminiscing about the old days when our High School Math teacher, Mr. Niles and his wife Gladys, who was our English teacher, walked in. I never thought I would see either of them again. I got up to shake hands.

"Hello ornery." Mrs. Niles said.

"Wait a moment. You're thinking about the old Larry. This is the new Larry you are looking at now."

"You had room for improvement." She said with a smile.

"It takes some of us a little longer to grow up than it does others." I said. I was careful not to end a sentence in a preposition, use a double negative or a dangling participle in her presence. She was always so precise in her grammar, as a good teacher should be.

Later, Gary agreed to show me where the Rest Rooms were. As we were going out the door, someone asked where we were going. "Gary and I are going out into the hall and conjugate a few verbs." I said loud enough for Mrs. Niles to hear. She still had the smile that one remembers through the years.

It seemed that most everyone had one of my books. I spent a lot of time that afternoon signing them for the ones that asked. Even Mr. Niles asked me to sign his. "Write something good." He said.

I don't recall what I wrote but I do remember he seemed satisfied when he looked at what I had written.

"You know, Mr. Niles, I spent a lot of time chatting with your wife a while ago. I want you to know she is just as sweet and lovely as she used to be." I said.

"I think so," he said.

"What have you been doing since retirement sir? I'll bet you are working on Fermot's last Theorem."

"Nothing that hard," he said.

"I don't believe you," I said. Something hard to do never bothered you before. If it were easy everyone would be doing it. Then what would become of people like you?"

I got no answer. He just smiled.

Later I ran across my old friend, Carl Broiller, in the hall. He greeted me with a handshake. "I read your book. Larry. A lot of other people did too." He went on to tell me that recently he had attended some function where one of the local ladies was leading the group in a prayer…"Forgive us our sins, dear Lord, and forgive Carl for offering Larry a drink of whiskey." Obviously referring to a passage in my book.

"Oh Carl, I am so sorry that I embarrassed you with what I wrote in the book. It was not my intention."

"Don't worry about it for one minute, Larry. You wrote it just the way it happened. Besides, I was here first; I was here before Moscow was even a town. As a matter of fact, I have Crown Royal for the dance tonight; you can have any part or all of it. Just in case you want to write another Book."

"Still can't drink, Carl. I am still on the mediation, but it is obvious you are still a man of fine stature. If the day ever comes when I can drink, I promise it will be with you."

At the Banquet that night, I couldn't seem to tame my knife and fork, so I ended up eating a pork chop with my fingers. No one seemed to care. If anyone even looked, they didn't say anything. I made it through another social event without any problems.

We all went to the dance later that night. It was at the fire station. They had some tables set up outside on the driveway but an unusual thunderstorm came up and everyone had to move inside. I couldn't dance, but I must have talked to everyone in town. I must say I really enjoyed myself. Greeting old friends and meeting new ones. I didn't think there would be anyone left there that I would know.

21

My Brother's Funeral

I made one more trip to Kansas that fall. It was on a Saturday. My sister called to tell me that my brother was in the hospital. The doctors said that he wasn't going to make it and that if any of the family wanted to see him, not to wait too long.

"I can't drive that far, Lois. I'll see about chartering a plane." I said.

"There is no point, Larry…He won't last that long," she said.

I hung up the phone I didn't get it on the hook just right and the phone would not work any more Later that day she sent me a fax, telling me to put the phone back on the hook. She had been getting a busy signal since she talked to me earlier in the day.

I called her right away. She told that our brother was gone. Somehow I knew before she told me. I think when two people are as close as my sister and I; there is a form of communication that defies logic. A year or two ago, when her little granddaughter, Robin, got killed in an auto accident, I could tell something was wrong. I didn't know what it was but I couldn't sleep that night. I was up two or three times watching ESPN on the TV. I have never done that before or since. When I returned from the cafe that morning. Stella told me that I should call my sister. She had called while I was gone. I felt something was not right but I had no idea that it was something this terrible.

Later that day, I was talking to Sy, my brother-in-law, about my experience. I hope I never forget what he told me. "It is because there is so much love in this family, when one of us is hurting, the rest of us know it." It is still true today.

The service for Cecil, my brother, was going to be on Wednesday, plenty of time for me to get here. Stella would not let me drive. She got me airline reservations for early the next morning. I packed light. If I needed anything else, I would just go the store and buy it

Everything was great until we got to Oklahoma City. It was about noon. I found the plane I was to take to Kansas. It was when I was on board that the problems started. It seems one of the fuel gauges on the plane wouldn't work right. We sat there for three hours while they worked on the damned thing. About every half-hour they would get on the speaker and tell us we would be leaving in about ten minutes.

At three o'clock they said it couldn't be fixed right away and that we should get off and find another plane. No problem there. I found the next flight to Kansas and got on board. It looked like things were working out after all. While we taxied in the runway, the motors all died. They had to send for help to pull us back to the gate. "No emergency power for a restart, we will have to have that check out," the pilot said.

RESTART…the word triggered a memory from an era long time forgotten. It was during the Cold War, late fifties, before spy satellites. One of our duties was to over-fly the old Soviet Union, taking pictures of Missile Bases, test sites and especially road, to keep the maps up to date. When we had the photos we wanted or if we would be spotted, we would high tail it out of there. We called them "Weather Mission" and were most likely off course because of navigational errors.

On one such occasion, I was in an unarmed reconnaissance plane, flying out of one of our bases in Turkey, taking pictures of Missile Bases and roads in Armenia and Azerbaidzhan. To update roads on our maps was very important. Then I was scheduled to go on to the Caspian Sea, then south into the safety of Iran. When I say 'unarmed', I mean we couldn't have taken candy away from a baby.

We were using a Northrop F-89A Scorpion. It had two Allison j35-a-35 engines, yielding 7000 lbs. of thrust each with afterburners, tucked against the fuselage under a thin wing, with split-edge full span flaps lining the trailing edge out to wingtip fuel tanks. It had internal elevators, mass balances instead of the external type on older models. The F-89 had a wingspan of 56 feet, 53 feet 5 inches long and a height of 17 feet 8 inches. It held a little over 1600 gallons of fuel and had a top speed of 652 mph. although it was slightly under powered, in my view. It was chosen in favor of the newer, faster, and more powerful F-94, because of its' longer range. The afterburners in the F-89 could be used for brief moments of climb and dash, but used fuel so fast that it could be used only sparingly. However in some cases short bursts of power may be more important than range. They had also dispensed with the solid black paint, previously the night owl's uniform.

On this day there was a C-130 flying the border along Iraq and on into Iran, testing a new sophisticated Radar Jamming device. It had all of the latest state of the art Hughes electronic equipment with no less than 350 vacuum tubes, 6400 coils, condensers and resistors. The slower moving C-130 was supposed to jam the Russian Radar so we could over-fly without detection.

The Soviets were so concerned with security that it made their Missile Sites easily detected. Look for a good road, with no sharp turns, making it easy to turn a long truck carrying a missile, that ends up at a complex with a fence around it, then another fence around that, then another fence around all of that. You could bet that it was a Missile Site.

Deep inside the borders of Armenia, an hour of boredom was broken by the scan of the threat direction scope. A new device we were testing as well as the new E-11 autopilot. They had recently added the new "data link" receiver. Performance changed very little but now fitted into the SAGE system. (Semi-automatic ground control computers.) The new "Threat Direction Scope" was one of the first attempts at beyond visual capabilities.

"Radar Scan," I thought. "Shouldn't be, if the C-130 was doing its job." (as it happened that day, the jamming device was slightly off frequency.) My knees turned to jelly. I could see them ahead now. Two SAM'S (Surface to Air Missiles) had just lifted off ahead. One a couple of seconds behind the other. We called them flying telephone poles in those days. They were about 36 feet along and packed with 350 lbs. of high explosives and all kinds of shrapnel. Nor-mally, this plane would have been carrying the New FFAR air to air, called the Mighty Mouse Missile, but that day all I was carrying was cameras.

Okay, fifteen degrees nose up. Got to do the job and get a picture of those babies AND the launch site.

Then: Those babies are closing the gap fast. Wait; Wait, I was saying to myself. NOW, hard right and dive. A risky maneuver anytime but necessary. If the maneuver is quick enough and extreme enough, the Sam's can't keep up. The first Sam flew by on the left. "Where is the other one?" I looked at the scope. Right behind, it could not have made a turn that sharp. Got to be a third one I didn't see that one coming. Major screw up. "What is guiding that thing?" Still thinking the Radar was being jammed. "Must be a heat seeker." No counter mea-sures on board. No flares or chaff to launch. What to do? In cases like this your brain takes over for you. It does things automatically without having to think. Throttle back, cut the heat signature, take another hard right and dive under.

A bright flash filled the sky, pain in my head and right hand, roar of wind coming through a hole in the canopy. Must have had a proximity detonator. A piece of shrapnel had come through the canopy, through my helmet and into the back of my head. Something else had hit my hand. Another cluster hit the Map trays at my right elbow. There was enough confetti from the maps flying around the cockpit to make one think they were at a Bar Mitzvah. Blood was everywhere. My head could not have hurt worse if someone had hit it with a baseball bat. The roar of the wind coming through the holes in the canopy was deafening. Can't worry about that now. Ignore the pain. I have other problems.

It seems that your brain lets you do a hundred things at once and then when the crisis is over lets you forget those things at least for the moment, and concentrate on a whole list of new circumstances.

Too much throttle back, flame out, engines shut down. Another major screw up. Shut off all electronic equipment, turn on the emergency generator, throttle up, hit ignite. Nothing Hit it again…again. Damn it was cold. The blood was freezing on my head and hand. Down to 150 knots, She falls like a rock at 115. Ease that nose down and pick up some air speed. Another problem, get much lower and anti-aircraft guns become a significant problem.

"Light off, Light off, God Damn it." The plane was a mess. Must have a hundred holes in it. My leather glove looked like a mad dog had been chewing on it. Eject? Are you Crazy, Larry? Have all of your brains leaked out?" I said to myself. Only as a last resort. Not over the Soviet Union. No way. They took a dim view of their air space being violated. Narrow-minded as hell. Men had been lost over their territory before. They were never heard from again.

Hit the ignite button again. At last, power coming up. Seemed like an hour had passed. Was probably only a few seconds. Ease that power up and see if the plane will stay together for a little while longer. I checked for damage. Half the right flap was missing. That was going to be a problem, but not right now. I remember an old pilot telling me a year before. "Flaps are for recruits, the old salts don't need flaps." Hope he was right! Can't be too concerned about the integrity of the plane right now, nor the pain in my head and hand. My forefinger on my right hand was hanging…Almost cut off. Oh well, I hardly ever used it anyway. I was more worried about the pool of blood I was sitting in. Also that if they send up a Mig to intercept my ass has had it.

Head south and get down lower. Oxygen was becoming a problem. I was freezing. Windows were all icing up. My bet would be that the lenses on the camera were fogged over as well. They will have to use what I have now or someone will have to come back and do it all again. Must get into the mountain so Iraq. Then ease back to Turkey if the fuel holds out.

Didn't seem like I was going south. Instruments say yes. One of the hardest things for me to do was to put aside instincts and rely on the instruments. Any pilot that loses a horizon or some point of reference, such a flying at night or in clouds or fog that does not depend on his instruments will lose control within 3 minutes. That is what happened to the Kennedy boy, I'm betting. I was young then. Armor plated and bulletproof. Nothing can hurt me now. How stupid we were back then.

"Stay alert. Stay alert. You don't have to have the Distinguished Flying Cross to do some Distinguished Flying."

"Get the hell out of here" That is what was paramount at the moment!

I was back to today, at the airport In Oklahoma City. "Have I been dreaming? Everything seemed so real." I looked at my right hand. The scars are there. A bunch of them. I felt the back of my head. There is still a dent. This dream was real, very real.

People have asked me what Airline I was flying on that day in Oklahoma City. It would not be discrete to say. All I can tell you is that it was not a Foreign Airline. It was an "American Airline."

'Get the hell out of here'. That's a good idea. I had my carry on luggage in my hand, telling the stewardess, "Let me off, please. I have had just about all of this I can stand."

"We will have it checked out in jut a moment sir, if you will just relax."

"You know, you said the same thing 4 hours ago. I think I have had all the relaxing I can take for one day." I said. "If you will just let me off this thing, you can keep my ticket, keep my clothes. Keep everything. Just let me off." I was wringing wet with sweat. Several other passengers followed my lead. "We want off too, they said. She grudgingly opened the door and let us off. I supposed a person that did not now days would be arrested…since 9-11.

I went straight to HERTZ and asked the girl behind the counter if she had a car ready.

"What kind of car would you like?" she asked.

"I have a way to go. How about a big car? I don't want a little toy car unless that is all that is available"

"We have a Lincoln Town Car that they just brought up. Would that suit you?"

"That would be great. Where do I sign?" While she was getting the paperwork done, I went to a pay phone nearby and called Stella.

I told Stella what had just happened, asked her to call Lois and tell her I was driving from Oklahoma City and that I might not get there by tonight. That if I got tired, I would find a motel and rest a little while. Stella said that she would take care of that for me.

"If I ever get on another plane, I hope someone shoots me right between the eyes."

"I think I know how you feel." Stella said.

Once in the car and on the road, my thoughts cleared somewhat. I had to concentrate on the road the map and landmarks that I knew from long ago. I was somewhere in the panhandle of Oklahoma. It was getting dark and I was long since past being tired so I decided to stop for the night. My sister shouldn't be expecting me until morning anyway.

I checked into a motel without any problems. I took a shower and looked through my light luggage for clean socks and shorts. I put on my socks and boots and headed for the door. I was hungry and there had to be a cafe nearby. I had a feeling something was wrong. What? I opened the door to find the café.

Room key. That is what I am forgetting. I went back to find the key. It was on the TV. I tried to put it in my pocket. No pocket. I was naked as a JayBird except for my boots. That's the feeling I had that something was not right.

I found my shorts and pants. Did you ever try to put your pants on without taking off your shoes? The boots got stuck somewhere in the legs of the trousers. I finally got everything back off. To Hell with it. I went to bed. I'll eat tomorrow.

I awoke before dawn that next morning. I had a tough time finding a café that was open. The folks that live here have every bit of my sympathy. God must have built this part of the country on the seventh day. Then he rested.

I drove on to the little town where I grew up. I stopped the car and walked the two blocks of the business district. Up one side and back on the other. Things sure change. Did not see anyone that I knew. I went on to my sister's house some 30 miles further. No problems finding her house this time.

"Where did you stay last night?" she asked.

"Not sure, Somewhere in Oklahoma. I will know when I get the Motel bill." I said.

My older sister, Elsie was there. She had been there for several days. At least she got to see our brother before he died. No one seems to know exactly what to say in situation like this. Me included. Someone asked me how I was doing with the memory problems.

Good, I think. I sent off for one of those memory courses that you see on TV. Thought it might help me. I must have jotted down a wrong number though, because now I have a lot of real estate.

We all talked, laughed and cut up for awhile but soon the gravity of why we were all gathered there set in. I don't know what I did or said for the next day or two. I know I was somewhat depressed and sad.

We all rode together to my brother's house. A lot of people I didn't know were there. Later we all got dressed and went on down to the church. I couldn't tell you a word that was said at the Funeral Services. At the end, I remember walking out with my sisters to the casket. I stopped to say "Goodbye brother, I'll see you later." I blinked back the tears.

We followed the hearse to the graveyard. One of the pallbearers was our old friend. Carl Brollier. I don't remember who the others were. Sorry. They had another service there. Two, really. There was also a military service. Flag and everything. He saw a lot of action in the South Pacific during WWII. Through the Marianas, through Guam and on to Okinawa. Some of the bloodiest fights of the Pacific theater. He was there all the way.

Later, the townspeople fixed lunch for everyone that wanted to stay at the church kitchen. Several people came to me to say, 'how good' or 'how natural' or 'how peaceful' he looked. I know they were only trying to make us feel better, but he just looked DEAD to me. How 'good, natural or peaceful' can you look when you are dead?

Don't get the wrong notion about how I felt about my brother. I should have gotten down on my knees every day and thanked God for my good fortune in having Cecil for my brother. He was with me when I caught my first fish, when I shot my first Pheasant, Dove and quail. He went out of his way to make sure I had a car for my first date. A couple of extra bucks in my pocket for cokes and hamburgers afterward. He was the greatest brother a fellow could have had and I am going to miss him, but his time had come.

An old classmate of mine that I had not seen in a long time, Nancy Olinger, caught me outside. She had just had a book of poetry, TO SOOTH THE HEART, published. She gave me a copy. There was a poem about me in it. I felt honored. Anyone can write a book. You can even use words or language that makes the reader think that you are smarter than you are. But it takes something else, someone special to write a poem. Especially a whole book of them.

My brother's first girlfriend ever, Donna Traran, was there. Still a beautiful woman after all these years. She asked me to ride back to the house with her. Just the two of us. We had a chance to talk a little. She told me that she had loved him since she was 10 years old. It was just one of those things in life that didn't work out.

Back at the house, I had a chance to talk to Betty, my brother's wife. I told her that she must be a saint. I know that it was not easy looking after my brother all these years after he had that stroke. She hung right in there making life as pleasant for him as possible. She will have a special place for her in Heaven.

I stayed another couple of days after the Funeral. My two sisters and I just hung out, talking about the old days, looking through pictures and winding down.

Lois made my return reservations for me the night before I was due to go back to Louisiana. I had gotten over my Red Ass at the airline. It is about a 4-hour drive to Oklahoma City, so she made the reservation for around 4:00PM the next afternoon. I left early the next morning. Didn't want to rush and I wanted to stop at the graveyard where Nancy was and say 'hello' to her.

Seems like it always takes me a long time to find her grave. I guess if I went there every day it would be the same. I know the drive where she is buried, but I always drive past, for some reason. Her stuffed dog was still there. A little weather beaten, but still there. Must be near a year now…. Still there.

"Hi Nancy, I thought I would stop and talk a bit while I am here. I don't know when I will ever get out this way again. I suppose you know about my brother. Perhaps you have seen him. I don't know how it works where you are, but if you see him, take care of him. Show him around. A lot of our friends have died since you left, Nancy. There was Rusty, Jerry, our dear friend, Bobby from down the Bayou, Robin, Charlie. Gee, there have been a lot of them. I'm okay with it. I think it was their time, you know."

"I think a lot about what if it would have been me rather than you that died that day so long ago. I would have missed the pain of losing you. I would have missed this Alzheimer's thing. I would have also missed meeting some beautiful people. I moved in different circles since you left. I also wonder what did you miss. A lot of joy or a lot of pain? I like to think God took you because he wanted to save you from something more terrible than death."

"I have been pretty much of a loner since you left, Babe. I never needed anyone or depended upon anyone. I can't say that anymore. I don't have a chance alone. I can't make it through this Alzheimer's thing by myself. I need someone. I thought I had a soul mate with Stella. She has been distancing herself from me the past year. It is like I am a bother. I am not going to disparage her. She is a good friend. She finally has a life though. She is teaching some sort of Art class over at the University and that takes most of her time. I might add that she loves it."

"I have made up my mind though. When I get back to Louisiana, I am going to pack up my socks and move to the Cabin. The life there is a slower pace, among the hill people, than the Rat race I live in now. Either that or perhaps it is my time to go. l was talking to Dr. Strub just the other day. I told him that. He said, "Why does a person ever want to die?" I told him a person doesn't need a reason to die. He needs a reason to life. Right now, I can't think of one. That could change."

"Listen to me rave on. I am telling you all this like you don't already know. I reckon you know everything that is going on. We have a couple of grandsons, you know. Their names are Josh and Jarrod. Sweet little guys. Sure wish you could have met them. Rhonda showed me the Ultrasound picture just before Jarrod was born. They knew it was going to be a boy. I couldn't tell anything by looking at the picture though. It looked like a dirty windshield to me. What do you say? Baby, he looks just like his dad!"

"Well Nancy, got to be going now. I want to drop by and see my old friend, George Rosel. He is buried right over there. Not far from you. Then I am going to drop by your mama and daddy's house and visit with them for a while. Keep up the faith, Nancy, and I guess you know that until I see you again, I'll be loving you. You know, they should change the wedding vows from 'till death do us part'. It should read, 'I will love you forever'. The memories of you may fade. Sometimes I go crazy trying to remember what you look like. But the love stays. It is always there in the heart. What has it been now? Ten, fifteen years? It doesn't get any easier."

22

The Documentary

I made it back to the airport in Oklahoma City without much trouble then on to Louisiana. During the next few days, I quit the Drug study in New Orleans, packed up my things, bought a new Chevy pick-up and moved to the Cabin.

I was happy and sad. I had told Stella that she was welcome to come anytime. There was a lot to do here to keep me busy. I had nothing to do in Louisiana. Stella had sold all the tools, the lawn mower, even my old Cadillac Convertible. I built a fence around the property, had siding put on the cabin, a lot of painting and polishing. I talked to Stella every day or so. Either she would call me or I would call her.

One night about midnight the phone rang. I answered right away. There were just beeps on the thing. It took me a while to decide that it was a fax modem I was hearing. I plugged the fax machine in and waited for them to send again. In about 5 minutes it rang again. The fax picked it up and started printing. It was a message from Japan. A company called Office Boa. The producer's name was Daisuke Yamamoto. He and his crew wanted to come here and make a documentary film on my struggle with Alzheimer's disease.

My book had just come out in Japan and someone with his firm had read it and wanted to know more. Seems they don't know much about Alzheimer's in Japan. I faxed them right back and told them to come on. Anything I can do to further the cause of Alzheimer's disease, I would do in a heartbeat.

They were here within a couple of weeks. They had quite a crew with them. There was Yamamoto, Shigeru Yamagami, the location manager. Koji Tsunami, the cameraman, Masako Tachikawa, the sound engineer, and the only female with the crew. Gernot Schreck was the interpreter from Austria. They also had a driver, David West, from Baton Rouge.

They were a neat bunch of people. They brought all kinds of gifts for me. Candy from Austria, shoes from Japan, all kind of little things. They were here for about a month. Seems they always had a camera running. They must have taken around 200 hours of tape. They must have had a tough time oiling it down to a one-hour documentary.

There was a lot of stress for me. Everything I did, I had to do again and again. I know how the movie people feel when they have to do a lot of retakes. Even when I went to the post office, I had to do it again. Seems like I didn't do it right the first time. Or they didn't have film in the cameras. You might know I locked the keys in the car at the post office parking lot. It took me an hour to get back into the car.

They all loved the food here. Seems they always wanted to take a break to eat. We went everywhere to different restaurants, from Mexican food to steak houses to the Country Club. If they were busy with some part of the filming, the driver went to McDonalds and got a sack of hamburgers.

They wanted to talk to some doctors. They tried to get an appointment with Dr. Strub in New Orleans, but to no avail. I told them about Dr. Pham Liem over in Little Rock. I had never met him but I knew a lot about him from newspaper articles. He graduated from the University of Saigon in the early 70s at the top of his class. He is the Medical Director for the UAMS' Center for Alzheimer's Disease and Related Disorders. He was voted the best doctor in America, a listing of the top one percent of the physician in his field two years running by his peers. He splits his time between the John L. McClellan Memorial Veterans Hospital and University Hospital in Little Rock.

I gave them his phone number and they called right away. He couldn't have been more gracious when they told him about their project. He invited them all over to the Hospital and worked them in between all his appointments that day. They were able to gain a tremendous amount of knowledge. He showed them all of the tests, X-rays, MRIs and the like that it takes to determine a diagnosis.

They finished their project and all went back to Japan. I had grown fond of all of them and I really hated to see them go. Yamamoto taught me how to sign my name in Japanese. I didn't have the where-with-all to learn any of the language. About a month later, Yamagami sent me an E-mail to let me know that the documentary aired in Japan and got a real good reception. He said it took days to answer all of the phone calls He sent me a copy of the tape on a standard VHS. I thought it was great. I wish it could have been longer, but it covered all of the most important things that the viewers would want to know.

Yamamoto must have also sent a tape to Dr. Liem, because in a few days I got another E-mail from Yamamoto telling me that Dr. Liem had called them and told them to let me know that a lot of the problems that I was having was NOT due to the Alzheimer's problem. They said I should call Dr. Liem's office and make an appointment with him as soon as possible.

I did what they suggested that day. I got an appointment for later on in the week. When the day came, I asked my good friend, Karen to go over to Little Rock with me. I just don't trust myself to go far away from the cabin alone.

She said, "Sure, anytime."

We left early that day. Karen drove to the VA hospital. I really don't remember much about that day. I remember we stopped for coffee somewhere along the way. I had a whole day of tests that the Doctor wanted to run. I can't remember all of them, but I do remember that one was what they call a "Spectra Scan". It takes about an hour. Karen told me later that they were about half done with it and I got up off the table and walked out. They came running after me and put me back on the table. Everyone was mad at me because they had to start all over and they had other patients waiting for the machine. I guess I thought they were all done. She said we ate at the VA cafeteria at noon. I can't remember that at all. After a couple more tests and about a dozen blood tests, we were through at last.

Karen wanted to stay in the city that night. The Ladies Auxiliary of the VFW was having some function later that evening. She tried to get me a room at the Excelsior Hotel but they were all booked up. Clinton must have been in town that day. She said she would try to get a cot for me to stay in their room.

"Nope," I said. "I am not going to stay in a room with three or four ladies. I am going home."

She tried to talk me out of it but I insisted. I remember driving out of the parking lot. The next thing I remember is waking up in my bed the next morning. I had made it home okay but I remember nothing about the trip. I went out to have a look at the Caddy. There were no dents anywhere so I guess I didn't hit anything or anyone. What really scared me was when I opened the door to get all of my paper work there was two one hundred dollar bills laying on the front seat. I looked at my checkbook. All of my checks were still there so I must not have written a check. I don't think I had two hundred dollars with me. To this day, I don't know where they came from.

I have been doing a lot of strange things lately. One time I lost a whole weekend. One day it was Friday, the next thing I know it was Monday. I had a receipt in my pocket from a steak house in Oklahoma City. I remember nothing. Those sort so things really put the stress on a person.

I really can't go alone anymore. I must find someone to look after me. I call Karen. "Karen, I was wondering if you would go to work for me. To look after me, to see that I take a bath every day, take me where I need to go, eat right, take my medication, keep the house clean and take me to church on Sunday. I will pay you the going wage, Even more"

"I don't even have to think about it. Larry. I will take that job in a heart beat."

"Well maybe you should think about it for a while. Taking care of an Alzheimer's patient is not an easy row to hoe." I said.

"Look, I took care of my husband for a long time before he died. He had cancer and the last few months, he could not even get out of the bed. I think I have an idea of what it maybe like. Hopefully, you will have many years before you get bedfast."

"Okay then. When can you come to work?"

"I will give my; notice today. I can still come and check on you every day. I just won't be able to spend a lot of time. The only thing is my car. The transmission is giving me trouble and I don't know how much longer it will last."

"Then you don't have a problem. Take my Cadillac. It is getting to be a few years old, but it doesn't have many miles on it. I am sure it will last a few more years. If it goes to hell, we will get another one."

Dr. Liem's office called to make me another appointment. They had the results of all the tests back and he wanted to see me. We drove over together and went in to see him. He explained things better than any doctor I ever saw. He showed us the results of the Spectra Scan. The red where there was no activity in the brain and the blue where it was still working well. Or vie versa. I never could remember which was which. It seems the most of the damage in my brain appeared in the frontal lobe. About 30 percent showed no activity at all. Hell, I don't know how I am able to do anything at all.

A lot of my problems, such as balance, no feeling in my fingertips and such, things that he saw on the Japanese film, it seems were caused by nothing more than a lack of Vitamin B and B-12. He put me on the new Aricept for Alzheimer' and massive doses of B-12 and B complex as well as E. Within a couple of months, I quit staggering and the feeling returned in my feet and fingertips. I can button a shirt now or pick up a coin from a table without looking at it.

Sadly, the Aricept did not work at all. The test scores kept going down. "Not to worry." said Dr. Liem. "We have a plan B. There is a new drug just out. It has been used in the UK for a couple of years with good results. I am going to try you on that. It is called 'Exelon'. I am going to give you your first month's supply and if you tolerate that all right, we will double the strength next month."

It worked very well for me. My test scores kept going up and the Doctor kept increasing the dosage At 4.5 mgs bid, the pills started making me sick. He had to cut back to 3 mgs bid.

"If we can just keep you stable at this rate, there is a plan C. In two or three years, we hope to have a vaccine developed for this thing. It hasn't killed any rats or lawyers, yet," he said with a laugh.

"Do you need a test dummy? I will take a shot of it if there is one chance in a hundred it will work."

"Let's wait to see if they get it approved by the FDA first," he said.

"What in hell does the FDA know about it? They wouldn't know a pill from a broom handle." I said.

He didn't comment. He just smiled.

From what I gather, for the first time in history, there is hope for the Alzheimer's patient. There was so little information about the disease when I first got the diagnosis. Now there must be over a hundred books on the subject. There are many sites on the net as well. As I said before, there are chat rooms. Chat rooms for caregivers and chat rooms for patients. I chat with some patient most every day. They are from all over the U.S. There is Mary in Oklahoma City, Laura and Morris up in Montana, John and my old friend Diana from down in Florida, Chip and Matt, Lynne and Lynn Mina from all over North America and Peter over in England. Ben down in Dallas all the rest. They all give me a lot of encouragement.

23

Preacher?

The medication has still not helped me in tolerating dumb, stupid people. Or perhaps, I am changing some in my old age. I quit going to one church because of an Idiot preacher. I go to church to learn and for the peace of mind that it brings. One day a guest preacher, who must have weighed about 400 pounds, was disparaging Garth Brooks, because he said 'hell'. He mentioned, 'The Black Element', in our town and then slammed gay people. He was quick to point out that Homosexuality is a SIN according to Lev. 18:22 and cannot be tolerated under any circumstance.

I thought as I walked out of his sermon. "So is Gluttony, you fat son-of-a-bitch. It wouldn't hurt you to drop a hundred."

I thought back to my knowledge of the bible. "Is to eat shellfish less of an abomination?" Lev. 11:10, "How about working on the Sabbath?" Exodus 35:2. It clearly states that they should be put to death, Is he going to do this himself or should the whole town get together and stone them?" Lev. 24:10-16

"I got a haircut the other day, even thought this is expressly forbidden by Lev. 24:10-16. Further, I approached the altar of God although I have a defect in my sight. I admit that I wear glasses. Forbidden in Lev. 21:20. Is there any wiggle room here?"

"We all know from Lev. 11:6-8 that touching the skin of a dead pig makes us unclean. Can we still play football? And by the way, according Lev. 25:44, if you are going to buy yourself a slave, either male or female, you must purchase them from neighboring nations, wouldn't want anyone to get into trouble by buying one here in the U.S."

I must thank that Fat preacher for again reminding me that God's word is eternal and unchanging. I wish I had asked him one question though. I didn't know this was happening at the time. "When my wife and another man commit adultery, which is forbidden in Deut. 22:22, which clearly states that they should be stoned to death, must I do this myself or is this a community affair?" All of this makes me really worry about my mother and dad. They planted watermelons and corn in the same field, a clear violation of Lev. 19:19. I sure hope they don't go to hell for that. Oh yes, you CAN sell your daughter into slavery, as sanctioned in Exodus 21:7. What do you think you could get for her in today's money? Wow. It is just beyond my capability to understand.

In my view, anyone that hates blacks, Jews or gays, (or Garth Brooks), because of who they are, had better adjust their tuner or put a little tin foil on their rabbit ears, because they are not getting a clear signal. They are not Mensa members, I'm bettin. You couldn't pay me enough money to go back to that church or any other church that would exclude ANYONE. I was always taught that Jesus did not judge people. These slobs judge everyone that walks through the door.

I was telling Dr. Liem about those kinds of people and how it bothered me. He told me to just ignore them and go on. "You are above all of that. Consider the source," he said.

24

Fairfield Bay

I bought a house overlooking the lake in Fairfield Bay. The house had caught on fire and had extensive damage around the furnace area. I was able to buy it for a song. I reasoned that I should have a place to live that is closer to emergency equipment. The cabin is just too far out in the woods in case of an emergency. However, I will always keep the cabin for its stress relieving value. Karen helped with fixing the place, finding contractors electricians, plumbers, etc. and continue looking after me.

She worked tirelessly at picking out paint colors, tile for the bathroom, carpets and the like. She can put shingles on a roof before a cat can lick its' ass. Karen can do a lot of things. She is a lot of things. There are a lot of things she is not. Within six months, it was ready to move into. She did a fabulous job.

I have yet to decide how I feel about Fairfield Bay. Some say that it is the ultimate residential community. A lush Country Club with two golf courses lined with mansions in the heart of the Ozarks. There are no jails or hospitals in Fairfield Bay although it is full of Millionaires and OLD people. It is an elaborately protected community for the seriously rich, a very small island in a very small world. There are the real Millionaires and the play like Millionaires. The ones that look like they are worth a million but are two million in debt. The rules are different here or at least they seem to be and the people like it that way.

There are hideous scandals occasionally, savage fights over money, bizarre going on at the Racquet Club or some genuine outrage like a half-mad eight year old widow woman trying to hit on the twenty year old pool boy, but scandals pass like winter storms in Fairfield Bay, and no one has ever been locked up for degeneracy in this town. The community is very tight, connected to the real world by only one road, and deeply mistrustful of their neighbors, as a lost tribe in the Amazon would be of them.

The directors of the Community Club, the governing body at The Bay, like their privacy, and they have a powerful sense of turf. God has given them the wisdom; they feel to handle everyone's problems in their own way. There is nothing so warped and horrible that it can't be fixed, or at least tolerated, just as long as the money keeps flowing.

Lots of people live here, but not everybody in Fairfield Bay has influence. The difference is very important, a main fact of life for the people who live here, and few of them misunderstand it (at least not for long.) The penalty for forgetting your place can be swift and terrible. There is no place for Horatio Algers here in The Bay.

The very name FAIRFIELD BAY, long synonymous with wealth and aristocratic style, is becoming to be associated with berserk sleaziness, a place where animals are openly pampered and those that don't 'FIT IN' are treated like dirt. Then there are those who delight in gossip. Their vicious gossip repeated enough could change the locals' opinion on anyone.

You can go to the Country Club and sit at a table with people who are speaking three different languages and see someone at the bar with duct tape holding up his pants. As long as the money rolls in, Huh? What a place! Other than that, it is one of the most beautiful places I have ever seen.

25

Karen

I worry that Karen may be getting bored with me. That I am taking up too much of her time. What if she finds someone that she wants to spend the rest of her life with? What will I do then? I couldn't live with either of my kids. They have lives of their own. I am growing very fond of Karen. Having her around. In all the time I have known her, I have never heard her raise her voice. She is always calm and caring.

One day when I was telling her of my fears, she said, "Look Larry, I love you. Why don't we just get married and end all of this uncertainty for you?"

'WOW'. I couldn't believe it. I didn't say anything for a couple of months. I really thought it over. It was not a spur of the moment decision. One day I said, "Okay, if you haven't changed your mind, let's do it."

"First, let me tell you now I will always feel about Stella. She has awakened me to new understanding with each passing word of her wisdom. She has moved my soul to dance. You have known people like her, Karen. They come into our lives like the beautiful birds that sometimes perch on a tree limb outside your window. They sing for a while then fly away and we are never, ever, the same. She is that bright shining star that would soon burn out here in the mountains. She is not like us. I am glad she was a big part of my life for such a long time. She will always be very dear to me." I had to blink back the tears.

"I know how you feel, Larry. I would never tell you who your friends could be. You are a lucky person to have had such friends."

We got married a few days later. A decision I soon came to regret. But for a while I felt safe with Karen looking after me. She made sure that I keep active and do all of the things that I should be doing.

I went back to Dr. Liem just yesterday for a checkup. They always do what they call a mental status test before Dr. Liem sees me. I always hate those tests. I get by really well until I can't do a simple math problem on the test. It is sad for me because in school I took all of the math I could take. It was an easy A. I loved

97

math. I took Algebra, Geometry, Trig, and Calculus. I did very well in those sub-jects. Then I took them all again.

I remember when I was in the third grade, the teacher was taking me to task because of the unorthodox way that I did math. When I told her how I got the answer to a problem, she told me that I could not do it that way. Hell, it worked for me and a lot quicker than the way she was teaching.

She gave me a problem to do so I could learn to do math her way. "Take 1 and then add 2 then add 3 and so on till you get to 100; then tell me he answer. She started back to her desk.

"That would be 5 thousand and 50." I said.

"How could you have done that so quickly?"

"It's easy. Get everything you can into hundreds. Take 1 and 99, then 2 and 98, and so on till you get 49 and 51. You would then have fifty hundreds. Then you have 50 left over. Add all that together and you have five thousand and fifty." I was real proud of myself until she made me sit in the corner for an hour. That was then….

Dr. Liem said that despite my math problem, I am doing well on the medica-tion. He did not want to risk increasing the dosage again for fear it might make me sick. I asked him again, "Dr. did you not tell me, some time ago, that the head injury from the missile may have caused this problem in my brain?"

"There is no doubt in my mind. As you know. Dr. Sue Griffin has done exten-sive study on head injury and I have to agree with her. I don't think people believed me when I talked about Alzheimer's and head injury in the past. Now they are starting to listen. It is in your genes. You are predisposed. You seem to be doing great though. You are responding well to the Exelon where the Aricept did nothing to help you at all. Aricept works well with about 70 to 75 percent of my patients. However, neither is a panacea for the disease."

He showed me a scar about the size of a penny on his wrist. "See, I too have a scar from a piece of shrapnel."

"Oh Doctor, I am sorry, War is hell, Huh? Did you feel the dent in the back of my head?"

"Yes, to both questions."

26

Stage Five

Stage Five is probably the most heartbreaking of all. This is the stage where the patient has lost everything. The ability to talk, eat, walk, to do anything at all. This is the stage that is the stereotype for most of the documentaries you see on TV. Now it is not necessarily the ultimate end for the Alzheimer's patient as I have learned through the years that I have been affected. The research people have been working tirelessly to find a treatment for this disease. They are right on the edge. We just all pray and pray again that God guides their hands in their search. Funding is very important. There is simply not enough money to fund every project that is available.

On every talk show that I have been on, I am asked the same question over and over. "What is the most important thing a caregiver can do for his or her patient?"

My answer is always the same. "When your patient loses his cool and blows up over something, it is not aimed at you. Don't act as if what he has done is unforgivable. It is just frustration. A pat on the back or a hug can do wonders in bringing him back."

Laughter is always good medicine. I joke with people a lot. Sometimes I think they take my jokes too seriously. One day last summer, I was at the VFW in a Pool Tournament. I had lost my two games and I was out. I started to go home when a lady said to me, "You don't have to leave right now, Larry. It is not late. Look, it's still light outside."

"Oh, I had better be going. I still have to round up the herd." I said without emotion.

Karen told me later that the lady asked her, "How many cows does Larry have? What is the name of his ranch?"

Another time someone asked me what I had been doing. I told them; I have been going through the Obituaries making a last, then marking their names out of the phone book."

I think, for a moment, they believed me. "So this morning, folks, I have baled a hundred bales of hay, milked the goats, fed the hogs, put up a rick of firewood, put out grit for my gosling and had coffee with three of my neighbors. All before 8:00AM."

"Good-bye, My friends. May God bless you."

Epilogue

This is the one chapter that I hate to write. I am so embarrassed. I have told you everything about my life so far, so I cannot hold back now. I think it will show you how judgment fails. How I could have been so wrong about a person. I can't blame this error on anyone else. I did it all myself. It is about my wife, Karen. You know the one that was going to look after me for the rest of my life. It seems that Karen has had second thoughts.

It all started when I got a note in the mail. It stated that: They thought I ought to know that his name is Jerry and gave the phone number and address. They also said to 'Watch Out'. It really scared me. I thought a total stranger was threatening me with bodily harm.I awoke Karen. It was about 7 in the morning. "I have got to goout to the cabin, baby, and find a phone number."

"What is all of this about?" she asked. I let her read the note after some arguing. She read it and said, "This is nothing, don't worry about a note that is just signed, A FRIEND." But I was scared. I went out to the cabin, found the number and called anyway. I called an old friend of mine who looks into these sorts of things. I read him the note and he told me, "Larry, except in very rare cases, you have nothing to fear from a total stranger. It is your friends that you know and respect that you should fear greatly. I will look into it a little bit though. Quit worrying." He had put my mind at ease somewhat and I felt a little better.

When I returned home, Karen met me at the door. "Where have you been for four hours?"

Didn't I tell you that I had to find a number and make a phone call? I had to wait till he returned the call."

"Well, I did some checking too. This is not about you. It is about me. They had the phone number and the address right on your note but the name was wrong. It is about Jerry Manzer, you know the guy I introduced to you at the VFW. It is just some more wild rumors. Someone probably saw me talking to him. The man's name on the note is the man that owns the condo where Jerry stay when he is in town."

"Well damn those busybodies. They sure cause us a lot of grief, huh?" I didn't have a clue that it would turn out to be more than that. Much, Much more.

"They sure do. It would just kill my Mother if she found out about this.I think you can just forget about the note." she said.

The next day, I opened my E-mail from my old friend where he states. "Larry, here is what I have been able to find out so far. Here is some E-mail between your wife and a fellow called Jerry Manzer in Michigan. Some photo attach-ments as well. Sorry old friend."

When I opened the attachments, I couldn't believe what I was seeing. There was a nude picture of my wife in a strange bed. It was subtitled, 'Coffee in Bed'. There was another of her still in the bed, title, 'My Phone Baby'. God I thought I was seeing things. This cannot be. I looked closer at the shots. I could tell they were recent. I read more of the e-mail. Jerry had states in one of them, "Thanks for last week. I never had so much fun in my life." I was devastated. I didn't know what to do. I didn't sleep at all that night. I finally got up the courage to say something to Karen the next morning.

I asked her what in the world was going on between her and her friend Jerry from the VFW. She asked, "What in the world are you talking about?"

"Please don't insult what little intelligence I have left Karen. I have it all. The photos he took of you in his bed. A stack of e-mail between you two. It spells it out petty well. Have you been having sex with him?"

"NO. LARRY. I didn't 'have SEX' with him. We made LOVE." (She used the street vernacular for 'Having Sex')

"Oh really. You 'Made Love'. God, I didn't know that. That makes it okay, Right? What happened to the promise that we made together that said, "I will love, honor, and forsake all others, till death?"

"I broke it," she said.

"I can't believe you did that, Karen. Not while we are still married. I had no idea that you were that unhappy. Couldn't you have at least waited till you got a divorce? The late night phone calls when you came and closed the bedroom door is making sense now. I just thought you were talking to your sister in Arizona and didn't want to wake me. How long were you going to keep up this affair before you told me or before I found out?"

"I was going to tell you about it after I got back from the VFW National Con-vention. Then I was going to ask you for a divorce…How long do you think this has been going on anyway?"

"I don't know. Maybe a month?"

She just laughed like I was the most stupid man in the world. "A year, Larry. A year." I do remember a couple of months ago when she told me she was going to Conway to spend the night with her daughter. Maybe go to a movie. I had noticed that every time I walked into the VFW, that she would be sitting next to Jerry talking. He was there every night. On the night that she went to Conway, I stopped at the VFW to talk to John Cook. I was going to go out to check on the cabin. John has said earlier that he would like to go out with me sometime and see the place. John and another fellow were all the people in there that night. Jerry was missing. Don't know if that means anything or not? He was there every night before and after that night. Makes me wonder now. *Your friends you should fear greatly.*

Further: I can now remember Karen telling me that she was talking to her mother awhile back and she said he mother had been asked. "Who is the fellow Karen is fooling around with?" Karen told me about that conversation with her mother. How they speculated on who could have started such a rumor. Rumor indeed. We thought someone saw me with my cousin, Johnny at Karaoke one night. You know people just love to talk and start rumors.

She said, "Then there was another time when someone asked her who I was having Breakfast with over in Clinton after the VFW closed. That was Sully. That was three years ago. Long before we got married. I haven't had Breakfast with anyone over there since then.

I agreed with her. That it was small town gossip…God, What a Liar.

"Well, I guess I have no choice now. You can have a divorce as soon as you sign back to me all of the property that I have put I your and my name."

"Are you crazy? I am not going to do that. I am not going to give up my home."

"You may not have a choice. I signed the property into both of our names because you told me that if I did, you would take care of me the rest of my life. You have perpetrated a fraud, Karen. You know little about Arkansas State law where it states: Community Property will be split 50-50. That is without fraud. We will just have to let a Judge decide that one. I can stack up witnesses from here to Little Rock that will tell the Court that the only reason that I put the house in your name too, is that you promised to take care of me. You are now breaking that promise as well."

"Well, I am not going to give up my house. I have done a lot of work on it," she said flatly.

"Didn't you think of the consequences when you "MADE LOVE' to that bastard? He can't be a very honorable man to put you into that position, a position where you might lose everything. And I will bet the VFW will be mighty proud of you. Having a woman like you as the District President. Nude photos of you all over the internet!

"He is a good person, Larry. He listens to me and doesn't interrupt me when I talk. He just sits and listens. He is a good person and so am I."

Right Karen, good people throw Alzheimer's patients out of their own homes all the time. Where am I going to go? Who is going to look after me? You have told me a hundred times that I would be dead by now if not for your care, that I can't stay at the cabin alone anymore and you are right. I can't cook. I burn myself all the time. There is no heat or Air Conditioning out there. I don't know if I can stand any more good people like you and Jerry. This is one for the Courts to decide."

"You mean you are going to drag all this dirty laundry into the courts, where everyone in town will know about it?"

"When it comes to my house and my pride, I will. I haven't done anything wrong except maybe buying your BS like it was on sale at Wal-Mart, staying at home alone while you stay at the VFW till it closes 4 or 5 nights a week. I guess I should have stayed there with you. You always told me that you were just talking to Connie, the bartender, or Karen Smorals, The State President of the VFW, talking business, you said. It appears that you were talking more than business with this Jerry fellow. You bet your life I am going to fight I don't think I could stand having you in this house and MAKING LOVE to anyone. I owned this house long before we got married. I can't let that happen."

I changed the beneficiaries on my life insurance policies and took all of the money out of the bank. I don't know that she would have taken anything, but in my view, anyone that will lie to you will steal from you. *Your friends you should fear greatly.*

I recall the night I called Stella and told her that Karen was going to be looking after me and my welfare. "You are making a big mistake, Larry. You know the things I have been told about her. Surely you can find someone else with better values than her."

"Oh, no. Stell. You are wrong about her. You believe shat everyone says about her. I don't think it is true. Just wait. Time will tell."

Right, Larry, Time will tell," she said. That is the last thing she ever said to me. Boy was she ever right.

How could I have ever been so wrong about Karen? I can recall back when Karen was working for me. Cleaning house, cooking, etc. I reckoned that she would not stay long because of this disease and the way it affects me at times. Even Stella was distancing herself from me. I think I wrote earlier in the book where Karen asked, "Why don't we just get married then, Larry and you won't have to worry about it?"

Right.

I tell you now. Normal people just don't understand the Alzheimer's patient. No matter how much you write talk, give speeches at conventions, they still don't understand. They say they do, but exhibit some of the characteristics of an Alzheimer's patient and they come undone like a two-dollar suitcase.

Karen said to me after all of this happened. "You don't talk to me anymore, Larry. When you do, it is just war stories of something that has happened long ago." Well, pardon me all to hell. That is all I can think of to talk about most of the time. Now I am being punished for it. It is odd to me that most folks understand people with Cancer, MD, Parkinson's disease and other horrible diseases, but with this disease where you look so healthy and are just sick in the head, they don't understand why you don't act like them. You wouldn't ask a person with no arms to drive down to the store and get a loaf of bread, but never understand why an Alzheimer's patient can not talk about something that happened yesterday or why he uses words that might be out of context.

"Karen, I tried to tell you about this disease, how it was going to be. I showed you everything that I had that was taped from TV shows or programs on the subject. I wrote a book on the subject that you have read. I have done everything I could to educate you about Alzheimer's. You said you could take it and wanted to get married anyway. You said that you loved me. In spite of all of this, I guess I will always love you too, in a very special way."

I know Larry, but I didn't know it was going to be this bad."

"For better or worse, Karen. That is what you took a sacred vow to do. Forsaking all others, remember? I guess I took it more serious than you did."

"Well, you abused me, Larry."

"Really, How? When?"

"You said I was hateful."

"By God, you were hateful. You haven't said a decent word to me in months."

"Yes I have. You just don't remember." (*That is getting to be a stock answer for everything. Funny how folks know about memory problems in the Alzheimer's patient when it suits them.*). "And you cuss too much."

"So do you, Baby Doll. You are as bad as a sailor. And don't you think you might have a drinking problem? You drink more than anyone should. The top-dollar drinks at the VFW. Is that really necessary? What are you trying to prove? That you have Class? I drink a coke or a beer every couple of months. Anything else bothering you?"

"Yes. You bought me a box of Candy for Valentine's Day. You said you were in Wal-Mart and saw the display so you bought them and gave them to me. That was two days before Valentine's Day and you didn't even take me out for dinner on that day," she said.

Well, pardon me all to Hell. Would it have killed you to tell me it was Valentine's Day and that we should go out for dinner? I don't even know the date today. I know it is August, but I don't know the date."

"You would have just said that you didn't have any money."

"I do try to be frugal, Karen, but on a special occasion, we could manage; even if we have to put it on a credit card. I do know that I have dropped twenty thousand dollars that was in the Money Market account in the last year. I can't do that many more years."

"I just can't do this anymore. With my mother being sick and having to look after her and you as well, there is just too much stress."

"One thing I do understand is stress," I said, "You ought to stand behind these eyeballs for a day. Only, I can't quit. I can't even take a day off. Perhaps you can go out and MAKE LOVE to some bastard you find sitting on a bar stool, stay out half the night and try to make believe that it is all right, but it is wrong, Karen."

"Wrong, wrong, wrong. I could not do that. I wouldn't do that. I may be sick in the head but I still have a sense of right and wrong. I have still morals. I can't say that about you."

She didn't say anything. Then: "This is my house Larry. I am not going to leave."

"That is where you are wrong, Baby Doll. This house belongs to a Trust. It is not yours and it is not mine. I can enjoy the fruits of the property, but not the property itself." It went right over her head. "The Trustee has been instructed to give it to you, IF you took care of me until I died. Look. all of this arguing is getting us nowhere. I am going to the Cabin where I can think. One more thing you might think about. If this Jerry Manzer fellow, the lying, thieving, slim, son-of-a-bitch, would do this to his wife, he will do it to you. A fellow veteran, too. May posterity forget that he was my countryman."

"If you are going to stay at the cabin while I am gone to the convention, take this food from the fridge out there with you. Be sure to eat it. It will spoil before I get back, she said. She loaded me up with several bowls of leftovers. "Be sure to eat this one, Larry. It is a tuna casserole with cheese on it, the way you like it. When I get back from the Convention we will talk. Okay?"

"Okay," I said. I gathered up a few things and my dog, Nell, and went to the cabin.

Let me tell you abut the Tuna Casserole. I spent the next day or two mowing grass, cleaning up around, polishing, etc. One evening I decided to eat some of the Tuna. it didn't taste good to me so rather than waste it, I gave it to the dog. My Nell dog is a Big Dog. She will eat anything. She is an Anitolian Karbash. She weights about 130 pounds. There was another little puppy in the yard as well as Nell. Seems there is always a stray dog around here. I split the food between the two dogs. The next morning, the puppy was dead and my Nell dog was sick for three days.

Salmonella? Perhaps. I don't think so I am just stating the facts and you can draw your own conclusion, just like I did. I am not accusing anyone of anything. However, I did report it to the Sheriff's department. They took a statement from me and put it on file. In case something happened to me, they said. One more thing that is suspicious to me. Since I am away from Karen's aegis, I am feeling much better. I don't have the headaches, upset stomach, and I can walk again without staggering. Again, you can draw your own conclusion. I did.

Perhaps you should read some of the E-mail I received. There are the first ones I received. There were more later. I will explain later how I got them I don't really know how to scan the e-mails into this forum so I will just copy them, word for word, I do certify that they are a true and exact reproduction under penalty of perjury.

Number one, as follows:

Date: Wed, 8 Aug 2001 14:32

From: Jerry Manzer<supermanz 72044@yahoo.com>
Subject: MISSING YOU....
To: Karen Zullo karenlee72088@yahoo.com

Just got all your Messages, Whew!!!!. I loved them. I don't know what my calling you at the Post has to do with the note to Larry, but I will respect your wishes. One of the things I didn't tell you was I got a new phone card from Sams for 1000 Minutes. Guess I won't call 3385 with it. I took, "Ass Hole" to the airport this afternoons and dropped her off/don't have any idea how long she is staying down there, and don't care. Got rid of Lucky (my dog) to the Amish in Mio the other day. I will download the pictures and sent them to you soon. Thanx for last week, I can't remember when I've had so much fun.

The next three are all dated Wed, 08 Aug 2001. They are all photos that he said he would send soon. The first one is Karen, nude in a bed with the caption: *MY BABY*. The next is of Karen sitting on a sofa, semi-nude, holding only a little towel over her front, with a telephone in her hand. The caption: *PHONE CHILD*. The third is of Karen sitting at a table with the caption: *LOVE THAT SMILE....*

Date: Thr, 9 Aug 2001 04:22

From: Jerry Manzer supermanz 72044@yahoo.com
Subject: NO COFFEE IN BED??????
TO: Karen Zullo<karenlee72088@yahoo.com

Thanx for the e-mails, I get so worried about you and that situation. Sometimes I think it would be better if I didn't come around or call or anything, bet its too late now. I "Love to".

She was going to leaven the dog, and I didn't want to be tied down that much, I know those people and they have little kids that will appreciate him a lot more that I could have. I'm going to call Lezlie when I'm done on this thing. (Daughter in Fla.) I have got horseshoes tonight and I will call the post from there. Please be careful and remember "Someone in Michigan Loves you very much"

XOXOXOXOXOXOXOXOXOXOXOXOXOXOXOXOXOXOXOXOXOXOXOXOX

Jerry

Fri, 10 Aug 2001 20:24

From: Jerry Manzer<supermanz1@centurytel.net
To: karenlee72088@yahoo.com
Subject: T A L K?????

TALK IS CHEAP...I WANNA

MAKE LOVE.

LOVE YOU, Jerry

Date: Fri, 10 Aug 2001 03:43

From: Jerry Manzer supermanz72044@yahoo.com
Subject: GOOD MORNINH BABY!!!!!!!!!!!!!!!!!!!!!!!
To: Karen Zullo karenlee72088@yahoo.com

Thanx for being you...I enjoy talking to you every time I get the chance.(Jesse too). I've got the appraiser coming this morning for the house, around 9:00AM. Hope its real low...I got my new processor for this computer, but I don't know how to back up all my stuff, and load it yet. I think Kris and Scott, & grandkids are coming up this weekend, and my sister and her husband are coming to their place just down the road. My initiation to the Eagles is Tomorrow at 10:AM in Hale. Billy Bob and my friend Tom are supposed to be there to help celebrate. I'll take some pics.

I miss and Love ya,

Jerry

I had to talk to Karen about this one. When he mentioned Jessie (Karen's daughter) I had to say something, "Karen does Jessie know all about this affair with this Jerry guy?" I asked.

"Yes," she said.

"This is a hell of a thing to be teaching your daughter. That having an affair when you are married is okay?"

"Oh, she has been wanting me to leave you for a year." she said.

"Really, is this the same Jessie that broke the windshield out of my Cadillac and never said a word to me? The same Jessie that I loaned $600.00 so she could get out of jail for shoplifting? The one that promised that she would pay me back? I never got a dime from her. I guess a person will promise anything to get out of Jail. Is this the same Jessie that I gave my extra Microwave to just a week or so ago? You are really reaching her well."

Karen didn't say another word.

Now that Karen knows that I have her e-mail address, she changed it. Didn't do her any good. The next is as follows:

Date: Tue, 14 Aug 2001 20:25

From: Jerry Doggie doggie57us@yahoo.com
Subject: OOPS
To: Milo Gonzales linda72088@yahoo.com

I called 7:30pm, Guy answered, I hung up. Your deal....

—Milo Gonzalez<> wrote:
I don't think Heidi really understands, but I did tell her you said Hi Dee-cute!!!!!!!! It helps to talk to you. It's really pretty outside. My Jerry Fish is looking at me. He still guards my computer. I guess I should fire him-he didn't do so good last week did he? Hut he is cute!!! I can't wait for National Conven-

tion to be over, I'm getting worried about it. My Mon is good and the back line depends on her. Will I better get off-I don't like to tie up this in case Mom tries to call.

I Love ya,

Karen Lee

Date: Fri 17 Aug 2001 05:35

From: Milo Gonzalez
To: Jerry Doggie < Doggie57us@yahoo.com
Subject: funny!

What do you mean your worried about the other people? And we don't have a cell phone. Larry had one a while ago but he stopped it-it cost to much, it was 10 or 15 dollars a month for so many minutes. We'll be careful and take our time-were not going to be in a big hurry. We have plenty of time. You make sure you behave yourself while I'm gone. Work hard and keep real busy. Oh and don't forget to think about me all the time! You might miss me a whole lot too>

I love ya,

Karen Lee

Karen left the next day and went to the VFW National Convention. I believe she was gone for about a week.

A few days went by and I was served with a restraining order. I has to appear in Court on the following Monday. When the court session was over, I had made Karen look like a fool, her lawyer as well. The Judge found no basis for issuing a restraining order since there was NO spousal abuse. He said to Karen. "In fact you are the abusive one." She had to pay the court cost and later the Judge gave me temporary custody of the Lake House. Her whole family was pissed. She may call me a Son-of-a-Bitch, but she is going to have to do it 'Long distance'. I am out of here. My train is leaving the station.

Later that week, I got a call from a fellow that said he was a Private Detective and that he was looking for Karen Rose. I told him that I wasn't telling him a thing until I knew for sure who had hired him. He said that he was working for a

Lady whose husband was having the affair with Karen; I invited him to the cabin. "I have some emails that might interest your client." I told him.

When he arrived, around midnight, we called the lady in Michigan and she affirmed that he was indeed working for her,. I let him copy all the emails I had.

The next night when the phone rang, it was the lady from Michigan. "Does the name Ruthie Manzer mean anything to you?" She asked. It took a bit. She told me she was the woman whose husband was having the affair with Karen.

"And how is that working for you?" I asked.

"Not good!" She said. "I have been looking for you for a month. I traced a Trust of yours to Texas, but no phone number."

"Oh, that was a long time ago when I had that Trust; back when I was in business. I am not sure that Trust is valid anymore." I told her. "Did you try the Phone Book?" We talked for three hours. This same scenario went on most every night for a month, until she cane to Arkansas to her Lake House.

The day after she arrive and got settled in, she invited me over to meet face to face. We had chatted on the phone so much that we felt we knew each other. What a charming and lovely lady she was. It was hard for me to believe that her Husband was dumping her for Karen.

Again, we chatted for hours. She cooked dinner; we ate, and chatted more. It was near the time the terrorists had hit the Trade Center and the Pentagon. Everyone I knew was sad and MAD. I was no exception. I wanted to get back into the military again. But Hell, I am so old and obsolete that about all I could do is play the Bugle.

It wasn't long before I spotted her computer. I wondered if there were any more emails (from Karen) on it. Soon, I found several emails that Jerry forgot to delete. You see, Jerry was staying there in Ruthie's house while this affair was going on. Ruthie was in Jonesboro helping take care of her dad what was on his deathbed. Great guy, Huh?

The Emails that were on Ruthie's computer:

From: "Karen—" callkaren13@yahoo.com
To: "JERRY" supermanz@hypertech.net
Sent: Saturday, June 09,2001 7:45PM

I know we have a lot to think about. We also have one more day to talk on the computer. Please talk to me: Ask me the questions you said you still have, tell me the things you said you wanted to say. You don't have to look at me. You wont see my crying. If things work out for you and your wife, that's ok. I won't bother you or even bug you if you come into the club/I just need to know. I need to know that what we had wasn't just something to tide you over till your wife came home. The way you look at me I believe you care a lot. I love you and I don't want to chase you away. I want you to listen to a song for me=for you, by Michael Bolton. The song is: said I loved you, But I lied" then listen to "Can I touch you There" by Michael Bolton. I love these songs and have had them for years, I think of you now when I hear them. Im sorry, I don't want to make you feel bad or bother you. I will always remember "our night". I love you Always.

Karen Lee

Next:

From: "Karen—" callkaren13@yahoo.com
To: "Jerry" supermanz@hypertech.net
Sent: Saturday, June 09,2001 1:11PM

I don't know what is going to happen with us, I hope something, but I do know that I have to make a change with my life. I know I cant stand to live like this anymore. You made me feel so good about myself and about us that now when you are gone I feel so empty and alone-I don't know how to explain it. Im sorry I cried last night, I love you so much, and Im so afraid I wont see you again. Love you

Karen Lee

(Strange. She says she has to make a change, she can't live like this anymore but for the next two months she was still asking me to put the CD's and Life insurances policies into her name)

From: "Karen callkaren13@yahoo.com
To: "Jerry & Ruth supermanz@hypertech.net
Sent: Sunday, June 10,2001 6:37AM
Subject: Re: Everything....

Thank you: it is a good morning? I love it when you call me Baby! I guess Im glad she didn't kiss you, Im selfish" I love you Jerry! I see my Jerry Fish first thing in the morning and get a smile on my face just thinking about us. That's good. I know you have to go up North (Where its cold) and take care of business but I sure miss you already/I will get you the numbers in Little Rock as soon as possible and I will love talking to you for my birthday. That's a great way to start my day. I love you-have a good day (not too god without me) and think of me-at least once)

Karen Lee

—JERRY &RUTH supermanz@hypertech.net wrote:

Karen Lee, Good morning Baby,Thanz for the language info, (suthin)< Don't you ever think you were just "Something to do" (that hurts). You just don't understand yet. I miss and I Love you so very much. My Marriage had failed long before I met you. A good example: after being gone almost two weeks, there was no attempt to kiss (peck on cheek) even, no hug no nothing!!!!!And I didn't care. All she could say was I dyed my moustash to dark, and bitched about my suspected drinking and carousing. (Little does she know). Anyway "That's a failed relationship" and I don't want OURS to fail. When I get on line up north, I will check my Yahoo mail supermanz@yahoo.com for any messages you might have left for me. (I HOPE) I also would like to call you on your Birthday, In Little Rock. If I can if you get any info on where, or when, or number, please let me know. Baby, I will understand if you change the way you feel, or if things get BETTER for you, or anything, But you will have to let me know. All I know for sure, is ME.

LOVE AND MISS YOU MUCHLY

JERRY

One more:

From: "Karen—" callkaren13@yahoo.com
To: "Jerry" supermanz@hypertech.net
Sent: Sunday, June10, 2001 4:03PM

Please have a safe trip in the morning. I don't want anything to happen to you now that I have found you. I think about you all day long. The way you look at me is so great it makes me feel so good. But you do argue too much we will have to work on that-just kidding! I love you lots. I cant wait to feel your arms around me again. I can't wait to feel your arms around me again. I cant begin to tell you what that does to me. Mom and I had a long talk about you last night. I need you to come back for me! I need your Love. I Love You.

Karen Lee

So, almost a month before the July 4th holiday, it is clear to me that her mother knew about this affair. After the parade, about ten or twelve people came over to the Lake House for a cook-out. Charmaine, her mother was there as well. She spent the afternoon eating my food, patting me on the head and telling me what a great son-in-law I was. Knowing all the time that her daughter was having an affair outside the Marriage. God, what an AWFUL, EVIL person she is. As they say; 'The apple don't fall too far from the tree'.

I noticed in one of the court documents that she filed where she stated: "Larry doesn't like for some of my family to come to out house." She could not have been more right about that. I really don't want the dope smoking son of a bitches around me at all. Especially not in my house. Further, her son in law joined the Army then deserted after about a year of service. I will not have him in my house. Ever, under any circumstance.

Let me put a cherry on top of all of this. I am single. I don't have to be half of a couple to be happy. Although I have lots or problems living alone, I have a lot of friends that look after me. When the time comes, my kids hire someone. More than one of the people at church has programmed their phone numbers into my cell phone. In case I ever need help. Further, Officer Murphy Taylor. a police-man at Fairfield Bay, that I have coffee with now and then, gave me his card with his police department phone number as well as his home phone number on it. His statement to me was, "Keep this card on your visor and if you EVER get lost or disoriented as you have in the past, just call me or have someone call me and together we will get you home." This one person has changed my mind about Fairfield Bay. There are good folks everywhere. (as well as a few of the other kind.)

I have the house back. You know, the one that Karen said she wasn't going to give up? Well, she did. I gave her the convertible, a trailer house and three thousand bucks to settle everything. Not a bad deal for Her for just a year of marriage. The good part is that it is OVER.

Karen's paramour, Jerry, went back with his wife, Ruthie. Good, I guess. After what he put her through? There is no accounting for taste. Ruthie told me that Jerry sits in the house drinking beer and watching TV while she spends eight or ten hours a day taking care of the yard and garden. She comes in and fixes his dinner and brings it to him on a tray. They must be a riot to be around. Everyone is different, I suppose. I have a rule. Don't bring me a cup of coffee unless you are going to get one for yourself. I do not want anyone waiting on me as long as I can do it for myself.

If I can stay half way straight for a few more months, there is one more thing I have to do that is important to me and perhaps others with mental problems. I intend to lobby the State legislature to strengthen the laws that govern people that will take advantage of someone that is mentally impaired. I was once very good at lobbing. The proof was in the puddin. I got results. There are laws on the books now that make it a Class D felony. As follows: 5-27-229 (criminal statute) "It shall be unlawful for ANY person to solicit money or property from a person he knows or should have reason to know is an incompetent person or is a person with diminished Mental capacity and to cause that incompetent person or person with diminished mental capacity to voluntarily surrender money or property in order to profit or secure gain by taking unfair advantage of the person's incompetence or diminished mental capacity." The law seems pretty clear to me but without an advocate for mentally impaired people, NOBODY CARES. NOBODY! I have cancelled checks made out to Karen for well over $10,000.00 and the transfer of a deed to some property to her as well. This was long before we were married. To me a clear violation of the above statute. NOBODY CARES! I know one thing about myself; I would never seek out any person and write out a check for $10,000,00 or give them a house just because it was lots of fun to do.

Further, if you think a mentally impaired person is going to get any kind of break when he or she goes into the courts, then you still believe in the tooth fairy. It all depends on what the court wants. If you are picked for jury duty, they will kick you off in a heartbeat, but if you are a defendant in a lawsuit, you are held to the same standards as everyone else. It appears to me that most everything I said was challenged as 'not creditable'. If you don't remember, you are going to loose. AND, when your adversary's lawyer deliberately misleads the judge with statements that he knows are untrue, it should be a crime. Maybe it is, don't know. In my case it was obvious that nobody cares! Why the state has laws on the books that govern the abuse of mentally impaired persons and are never used is far beyond my ability to understand. Perhaps it is better in the bigger cities. Wasn't it Dennis Miller that said? "You can't get justice in any courtroom that uses a ceiling fan."

Among the frustrating, confusing and negative things that happen everyday, there are still a few things that happen that make life still worth living. I had the pleasure of meeting Dr. "Patch" Adams, the other day at an Alzheimer's conference in Tulsa. Moreover, I got to chitchat with him, one on one, for ten or fifteen minutes. What a remarkable man he is.

Then again, when I am sitting on the pity pot, I get a card like this:

Larry

We have known you for almost 6 years now. You have been a blessing for us from day one.

We have seen and heard of your life's examples of Faith. Not in you're carrying around a big Bible under your arm or quoting lots of scriptures but we see this in your heart and triumphing daily. We hear of your pastor, your church and friends.

We see your faith in action through your hands extended to others in love and in things you do and we hear. Like installing a new ceiling fan for a widow, or showing kindness and concern for a neighbor who doesn't come around for a couple of days and checking to see if they are okay.

We have seen you helping a handicapped person get in and out of his chair at the Senior Center or spreading his butter on a piece of bread and opening his container of milk while his wife is busy.

I have seen you help a 92 year old man better understand the complexities of a computer. And as we witness your explanation to others about your trials, we know God will continue to use this honesty about your experiences to make our faith strong and use you as an example to others who are suffering and feel all by themselves in trying times.

God truly is our refuge and strength and very, very present help in times of need, Larry. Keep smiling, keep writing your books. We are truly blessed by knowing you.

Frank and Jo Ann

I am at a loss for anything to say after reading a letter like this. But, it keeps me going another day. If one were to ask God "Why am I still here? Isn't my work done?" He would probably say. "If you are still alive, it isn't."

Just one more thing. I have a personal message for Karen. "If anyone ever offers you a breath mint. Take it."

Thanks everyone for reading my book. I love you all.

0-595-28927-4